Runic Mandalas

Path to Meditation and Healing

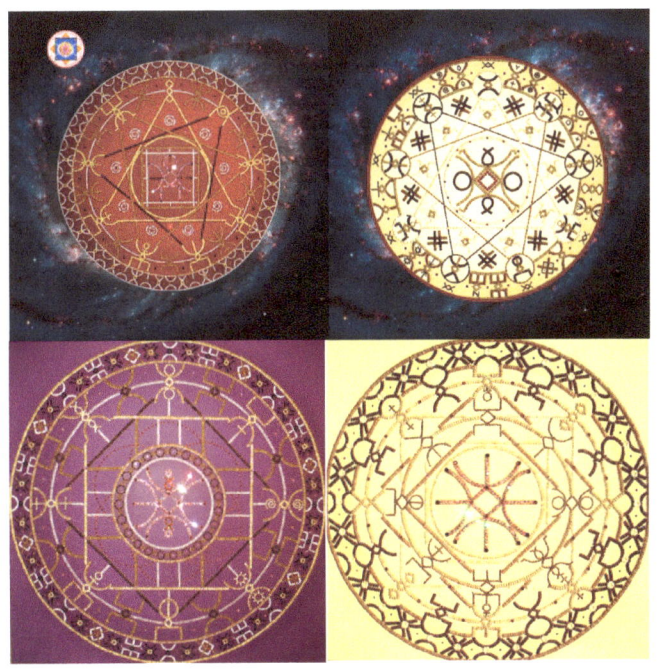

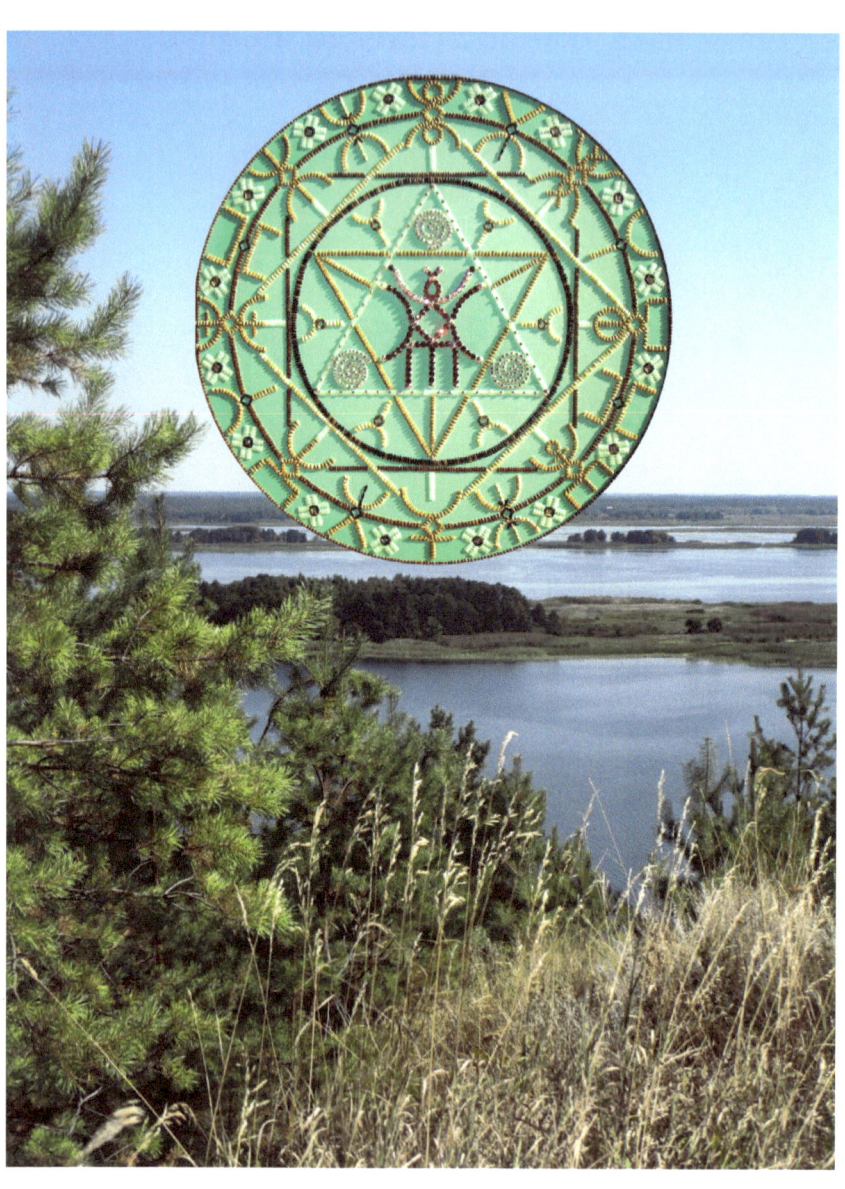

Runic Mandalas

Path to Meditation and Healing

Dr. Nadejda B. Matsko

CWP
Central West Publishing

For more information about the books published by Central West Publishing, please visit https://centralwestpublishing.com

Disclaimer
Every effort has been made by the publisher and author while preparing this book, however, no warranties are made regarding the accuracy and completeness of the content. The publisher and author disclaim without any limitation all warranties as well as any implied warranties about sales, along with fitness of the content for a particular purpose. Citation of any website and other information sources does not mean any endorsement from the publisher and author. For ascertaining the suitability of the contents contained herein for a particular lab or commercial use, consultation with the subject expert is needed. In addition, while using the information and methods contained herein, the practitioners and researchers need to be mindful for their own safety, along with the safety of others, including the professional parties and premises for whom they have professional responsibility. To the fullest extent of law, the publisher and author are not liable in all circumstances (special, incidental, and consequential) for any injury and/or damage to persons and property, along with any potential loss of profit and other commercial damages due to the use of any methods, products, guidelines, procedures contained in the material herein.

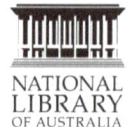 A catalogue record for this book is available from the National Library of Australia

ISBN (print): 978-1-925823-91-2

Contents

Preface

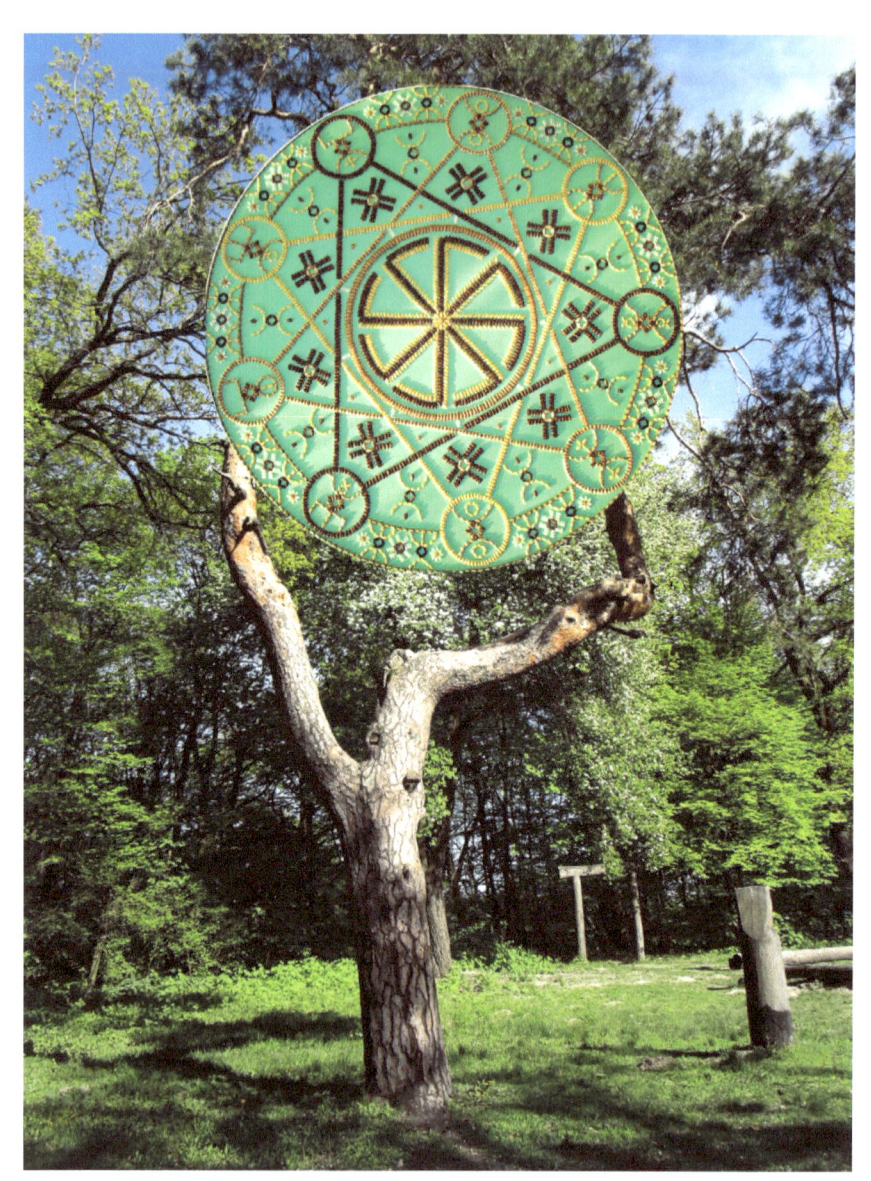

Preface

Touch and feel how you were touched,
plunging into the depths and feel the filling,
glide on the surface and see your reflection,
there is no justice, there are resonances in this world.

We strive for the best all our lives. At least consciously. No matter which difficult situation a person finds himself in, there is always a hope inside that there is a way out and that the world will turn out to be different. The wise say that there is no stronger opponent than a half-truth. One can always find a way out, and a lot of things can be changed, however, not by conquering the world using force or by endlessly waiting for things to turn out by themselves. I'm talking about the way to align with the desired and releasing the internal resource for its implementation. The life energy in its various manifestations (strength, chorism, finances, talents, etc.) is inherent in each of us by Nature just after birth. All that is necessary is to create the right conditions so that the energy can manifest itself. Here, almost everything lies in the hands of the person himself. If the inner spring of energy is littered with stones of previous traumas and negative experiences, there is no point in waiting for these stones to suddenly dissolve and fade away. Nor does it make sense to destroy them, thereby complicating the situation. It makes sense to gradually remove them layer by layer, until the energy is manifested in all its power and diversity. Most importantly, it is wonderful if one does it with pleasure, enjoying the process, and not postponing the life for later.

One can clear the internal space in a thousand different ways. Working with emotions, changing the thinking and physical practices that liberate the body are currently available and achievable. However, there are times when we do not have the initial resources and determination to ask for help. This is where independent work with runes, mandalas or any other approach based on the principle of resonance can come to the rescue. We align with the reference natural energies, such as Purification, Restoration, Prosperity and Love, concentrated in ancient symbols, and gradually our potential rises from the depths of our nature, resonating with these energies. We begin to "sound" in a new way, and the outside world turns to us with a new desired face. It is worth a try to attain the pleasure and find a new self free from the old shackles and restrictions. If the approach turns out to be yours, the movement will lead you to the path of free movement, growth and development, which almost every creature of the Nature strives for.

Nadejda B. Matsko
November 2020

1

Introduction

We absolutely must leave room for doubt or there is no progress and no learning. There is no learning without having to pose a question, and a question requires doubt. People search for certainty, but there *is* no certainty. People are terrified - how can you live *and not know*? It is not odd at all. You only think you know, as a matter of fact. Most of your actions are based on incomplete knowledge and you really don't know what it is all about, or what is the purpose of the world, or how a great deal of other things function. It is possible to live and not know. - **Richard Phillips Feynman**, Nobel laureate in quantum physics

Even being in the paradigm of classical science (collection of facts, systematization, critical analysis, etc.), we are forced to admit that there are areas of natural manifestations that so far cannot be comprehensively understood and adequately modeled. This is especially true for the description of the human brain and its regulatory functions. With a large number of existing models and theories, we are still not able to reliably predict what the next step will be, not to mention the experienced emotion of an individual. Moreover, the reason here is not only the dynamic and complex physiology making the available set of factors unable to decipher the full picture. Such manifestations as the generic and social unconsciousness come into play, the influence of which on physiology is practically not studied at all, although its presence has been proved.

However, despite the enormous complexity and versatility of the natural processes, a person, nevertheless, manages to maintain, develop and heal the vital activity of the body in the event of external and internal injuries, not only by resorting to the opportunities provided by the classical sciences, such as traditional physics, medicine, biology, cytology, etc., but also using methods completely far from the "calculated physical and chemical effects", such as the therapy of sound, color and touch as well as the therapy which uses sacred geometric symbols as a method of influencing our consciousness (mandala therapy, rune therapy, image and art therapy, etc.)

At this juncture, I do not intend to fully and accurately explain from a physical point of view why contactless therapy can be very effective. However, I wish to clarify several principles of contactless interaction between the human body and surrounding world that affect and change the physical characteristics of the human body.

"If you want to learn the secrets of the universe, think in units of energy, frequency and vibration", said a great physicist of our time, Nikola Tesla. We really live in a world where information comes to us in the form of vibrations. First of all, it is light. The color, visual volume and dimensions, brightness, etc., are the result of the interaction of the wave structures with the optical system of our eyes. The presence of two eyes allows us to create a stereo-image (volumetric) of the objects surrounding us and, thus, greatly facilitates the orientation in the surrounding space without sticks **(Illus. 1)**. With our ears, we pick up sound vibrations, also in the stereo-mode. However, the most important thing to remember is that the person himself is a complex oscillatory circuit, along with keeping in focus the material objects surrounding us: "living" in the sense of "green and moving" as well as "not living" stones, water, air and fire. Importantly, in any atom, the elementary particles are in continuous and fast movement. The modern science can measure femtosecond events at the maximum, however, there are much faster processes that constantly happen inside the atomic structure of the materials. The molecules are built from atoms, which also continuously move and vibrate due to not only the atomic vibrations, but also the chemical and electrostatic bonds binding these atoms. The connections serve as a kind of hinges with a certain number of degrees of freedom, i.e., the ability to "bend" right-to-left, compress-stretch, etc. **(Illus. 2)**. The molecular chains are built from molecules, such as, proteins, DNA, RNA, carbohydrates and fats. The organs are built from proteins and organisms from organs. Each molecular structure vibrates uninterruptedly, and the more complex is the structure, the greater is the number of processes occurring simultaneously in its depths. Based on this phenomenon, there are a large number of diagnostic devices that, for example, record the infrared spectrum of the vibrations of an organ and compare it with "averagely healthy characteristics", thus, revealing pathological issues in this way, if any.

If you look at a person as well as at the material world surrounding him from the point of view of "everything fluctuates", many mysterious influences and interactions consequently become understandable, such as, a person and a mineral, a person and an art, a person and a symbol, etc.

The fact is that each oscillatory circuit has several dominant internal frequencies that are characteristic of this particular oscillatory system. Accordingly, this is true for our body and for a stone lying on the road. Obviously, these frequencies are individual for each system, and as there are no two identical fingerprints, there are no two identical frequency profiles. For minerals, for example, the structure is often crystalline or polycrystalline (consisting of the segments of the amorphous and non-ordered matter interposed by the highly organized matter, such as crystals). The oscillations of such a formation are significantly different from the spectra of the living organisms **(Illus. 3)**. Consequently, the question remains: how do we interact with each other? In physics, two main paths of interaction are possible for the two oscillatory circuits. The first is simply the imposition of vibrations. Such an interaction does not change anything in the structure and response of the "participants". In everyday life, this type of interaction will correspond to the statement, "...but somehow I did not even notice". We can meet the same person hundreds of times on the street while going to work and ultimately never see him. There is a second type of interaction, which is known as **resonance**. In physical perspective, this is described as the phenomenon of a significant increment in the amplitude of the forced oscillations of the system, which occurs when the frequency of the external action approaches certain values (resonance frequencies) due to the properties of the system. Thus, the cause of resonance is the coincidence of the external (exciting) frequency with the internal (natural) frequency of the oscillatory system. Resonance is found in mechanics, electronics, optics, acoustics and astrophysics **(Illus. 4)**. In simplified language, this can be envisaged as a change in the internal state when interacting with something that has the frequency characteristics close to those we have inside. Moreover, we know a little about it until the moment of "significant meeting". This is how love happens at first sight, or antipathy at first breath. We can see almost ten identical ornaments, and suddenly one of them causes a clear internal response, "mine"!! The uniqueness of the resonant interactions is primarily characterized by the fact that they CHANGE something inside US. Moreover, some resonant interactions can have an obsessive and sometimes suppressive or addictive effect. Almost all alternative medicine and psychological practices lie in the field of resonant interactions. Unlike chemistry, which works without taking into account the individual characteristics of the body, "you are having a fever, take Aspirin", the resonance therapy is in turn tuned to a specific person and helps to change something in the person due to HIS OWN processes, arising as a response to an external action. As the mutual resonance is drained, the connection is interrupted. For instance, I would like to provide a visual experience known from the school days. We will consider two identical resonators, such as the ones usually used to tune the musical instruments. A small bead is fitted to the shoulder of one of the resonators. As we excite a sound in one of the resonators with a wooden stick to initiate it to start generation sound, the bead next to the second deviates and comes into an oscillatory motion **(Illus. 5)**. This suggests that the resonator, which no one touched with a finger, begins to spontaneously vibrate just at the same frequency as the mechanically excited one. If we change the structure of one of the resonators by attaching an additional load to one of the arms of the resonator fork and repeat the exact experiment, the bead will remain motionless **(Illus. 6)**. The modified resonator does not sound "in response." From this simple experiment, one can understand very many psychological features of the interactions between the people.

What usually attracts us to others is some of our own qualities, both constructive and destructive, which for some reason were not manifested externally until that time (due to psychological limitations, or lack of resources, or society not supporting such behavior). As we look deeply at the problem and allow the hidden to become apparent, the painful dependence on an external object disappears. The resonant interaction can also explain the fact that being close to a harmonious well-developed person, many problems are solved by themselves. I want to emphasize here that the harmonious and one-sided are not the same thing. Positivism in terms, "I am the best," more often indicates a significant pile of pain, long and securely hidden in the subconscious. Such a person exerts all his strength and will in order to appear to be someone he is not. A harmonious state gives place to all of its own manifestations, without suppressing anything and "not hiding anything under the carpet." Usually, such a person serves the healing of others simply by his presence.

Finally, the most significant aspect is that through internal resonances, if we pay attention to them, one can find inside the source of inexhaustible strength and energy. Our body knows much better than our conscious mind how to be healed. We may not remember how to take generic or natural (due to psychological trauma, broken connections, etc.) energy, however, our body knows how to and strives for it. Following the resonance without trying to find the logical answers and just trusting the process, we are able to help ourselves much more effectively. Thus, the key lies in not breaking our own nature to standards, but discovering and expressing all of its aspects. Intelligent is not the one who understands, but the one who knows how to correctly use his own potential.

Image Sources: *Illustrations were partially taken from sites* https://www.pexels.com/ *and* https://pxhere.com/ *(Creative Commons Zero (CC0) license).*

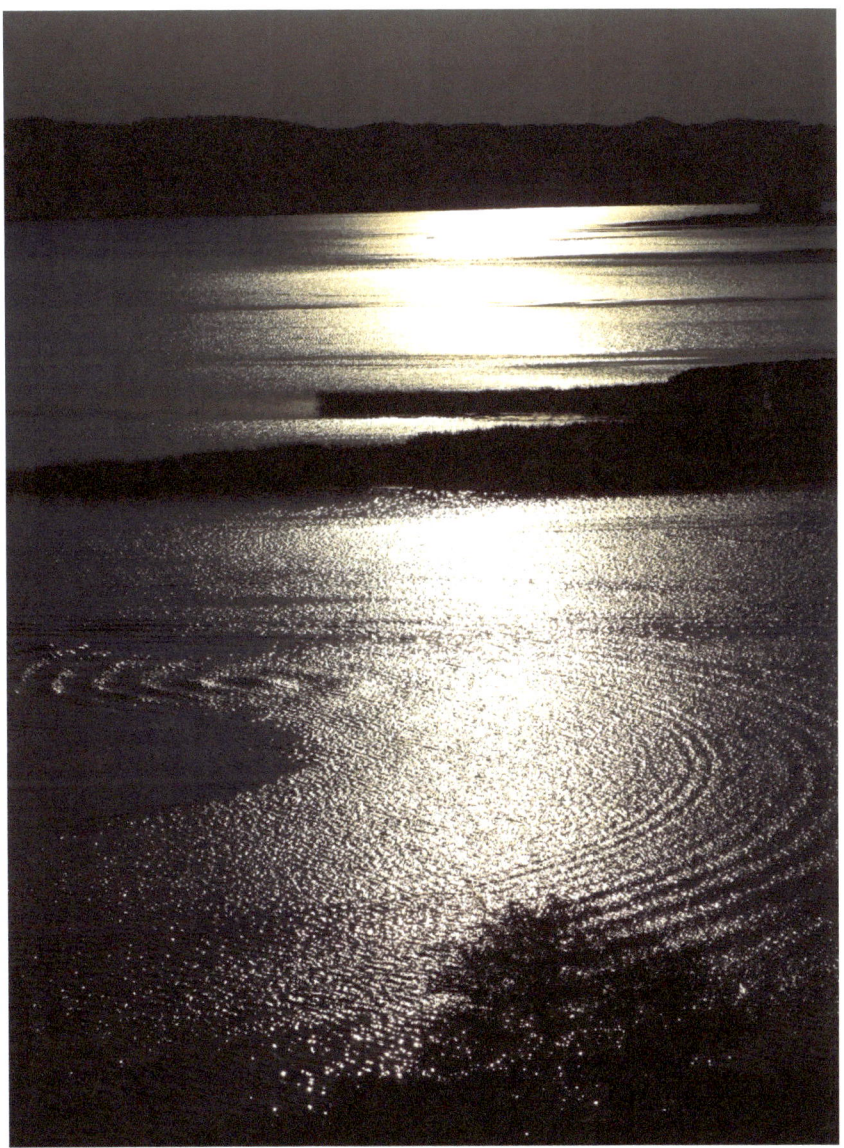

Illustration 1. *The oscillatory nature of water.*

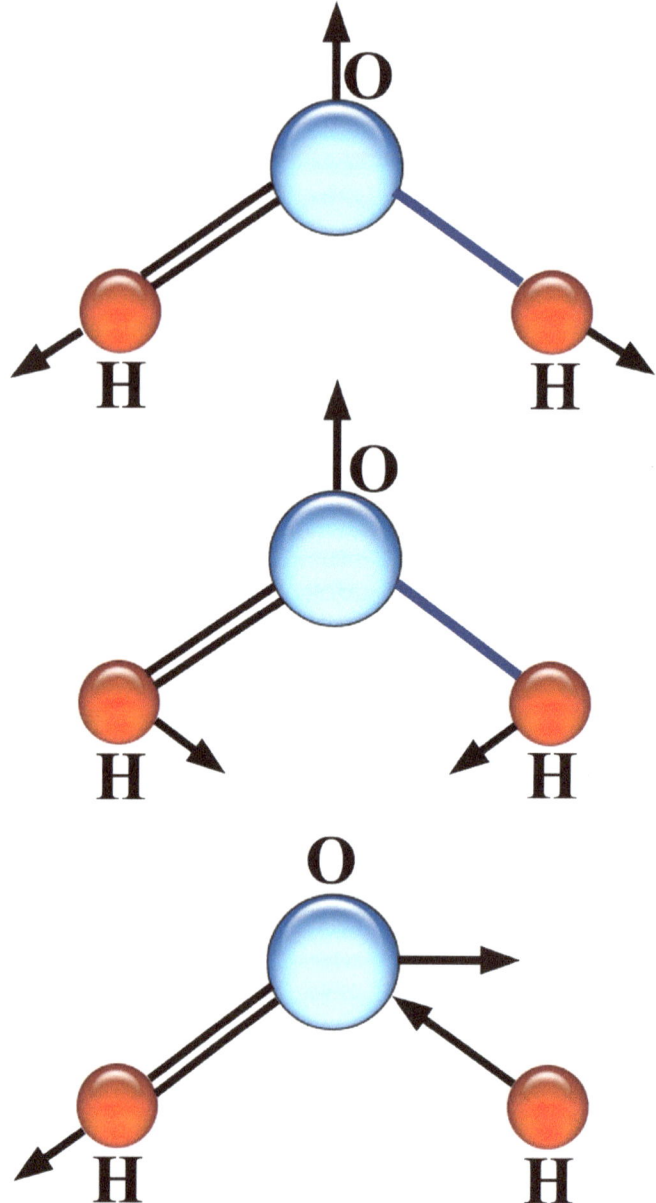

Illustration 2. *The vibrations of the water molecules. Due to the existing degrees of freedom of the molecular bonds, the atoms can move in several directions.*

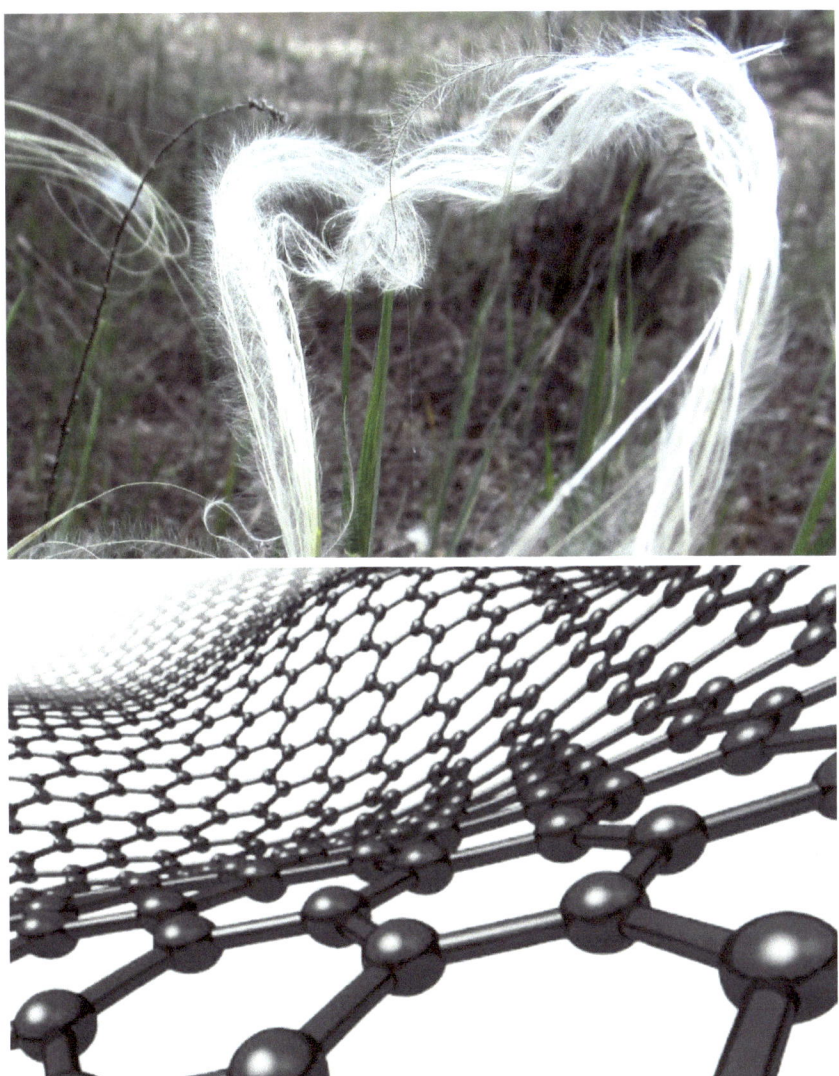

Illustration 3. *Natural vibrations of living organisms. Feather grass (top picture); and schematic representation of the thermal vibrations of the graphene crystal lattice (bottom picture).*

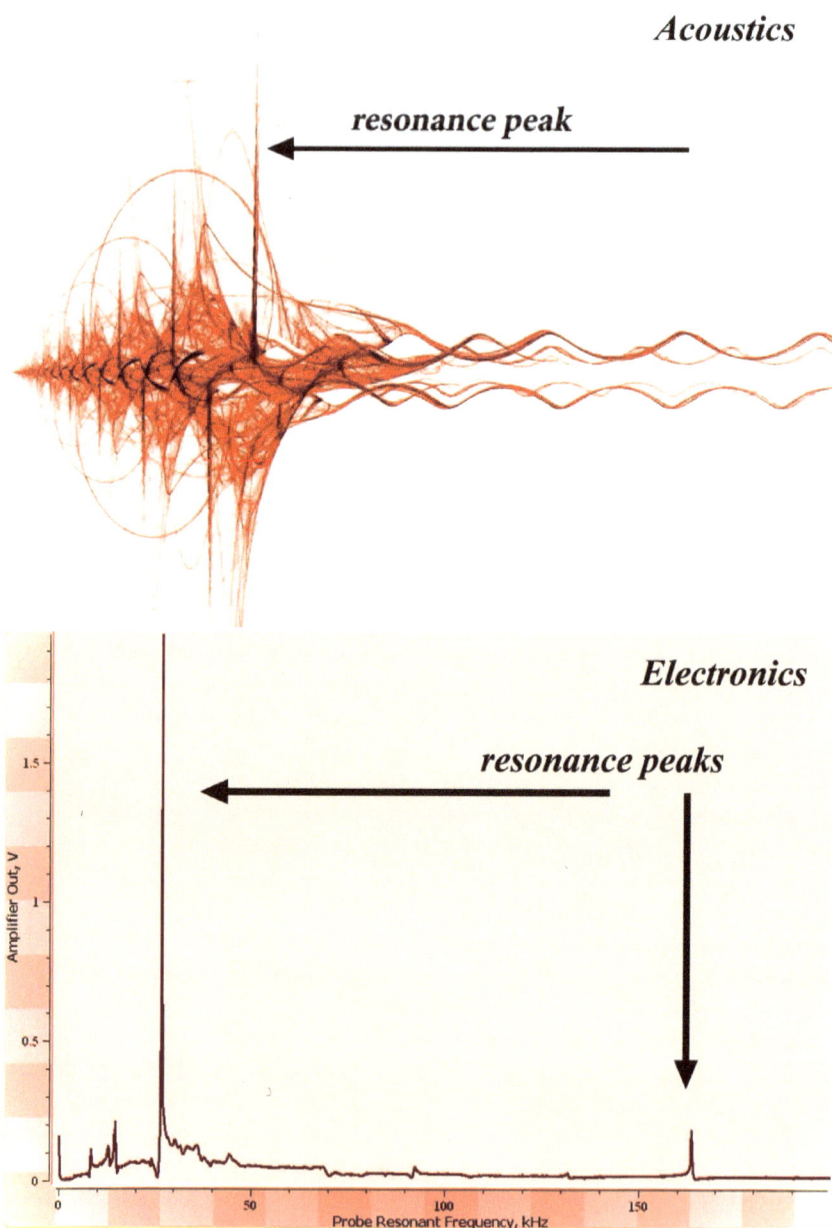

Illustration 4. *Resonance curves in different systems.*

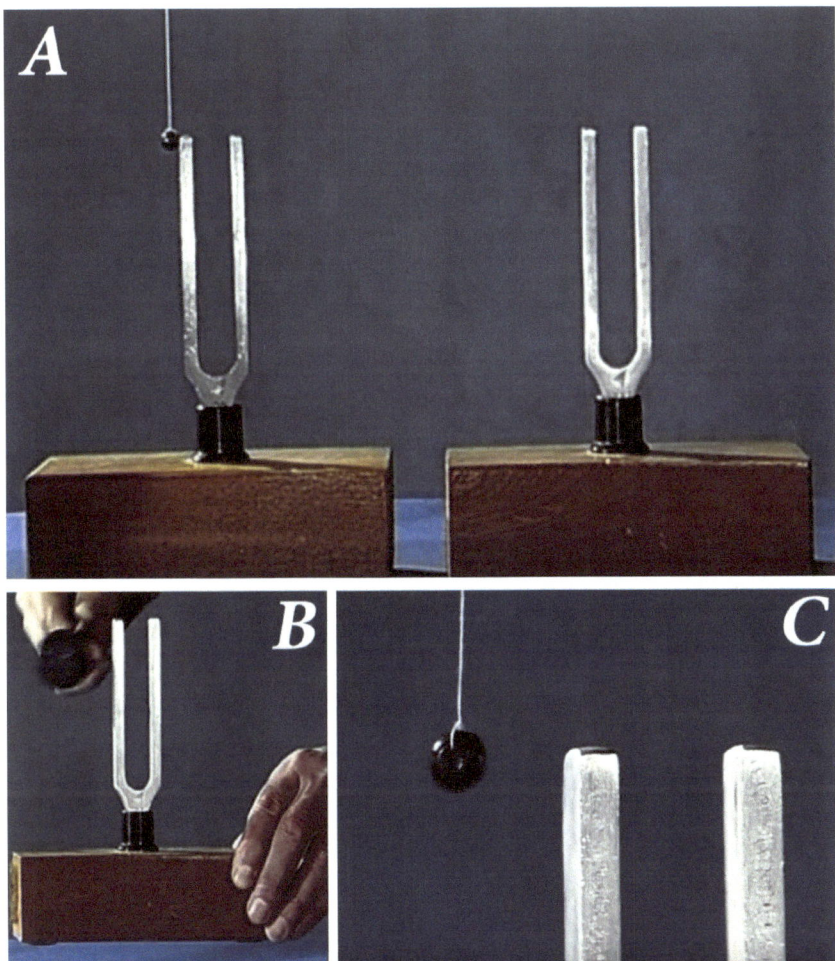

Illustration 5. *An experiment with two identical tuning forks mounted on the resonant boxes. A) Resonators are placed nearby. The shoulder of one of the resonators is touched by a bead attached to the strut, B) one of the tuning forks is struck with a wooden stick, and C) the bead adjacent to the tuning fork, which no one has touched, starts to bow and oscillate.*

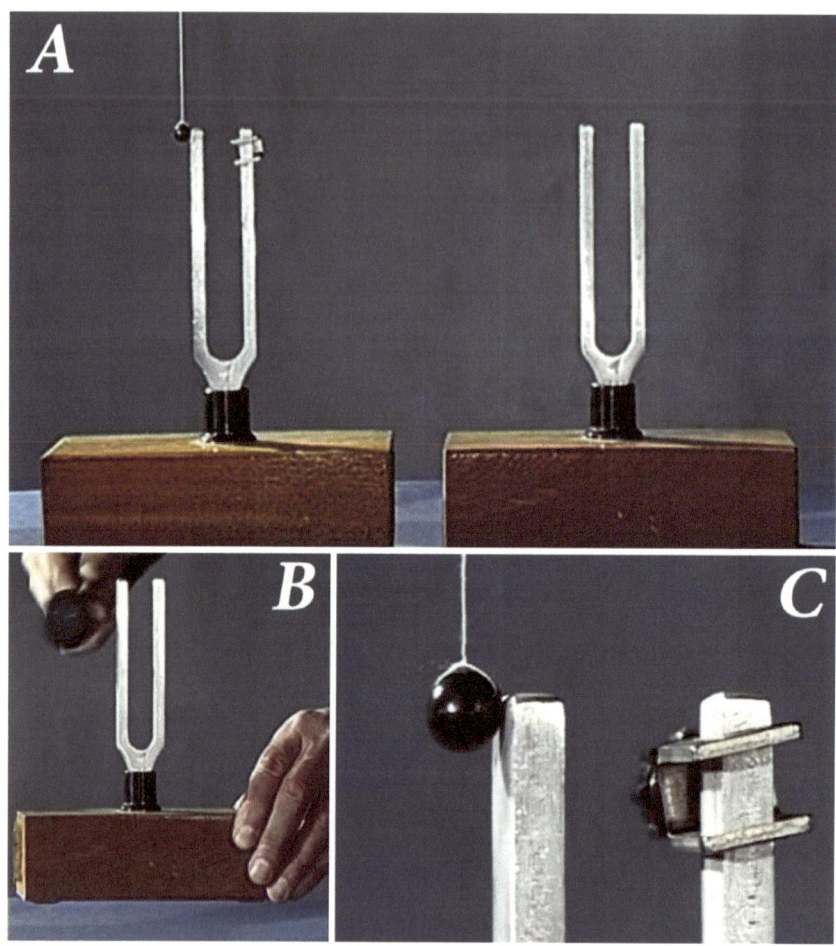

Illustration 6. *An experiment with two identical tuning forks mounted on the resonant boxes. An additional load is attached to the shoulder of one of the tuning forks. A) Resonators are placed nearby. The bead attached to the rack touches the shoulder of one of the resonators, B) one of the tuning forks is struck with a wooden stick, and C) the bead adjacent to the tuning fork with a load, which no one has touched, remains stationary.*

2

Mandala

The mandala is the oldest magic resonator. It acts both at the psy-chophysiological level, changing the electrical activity of the brain and at the level of psycho-energy, creating powerful informational biological fields. These fields can carry a protective, activating and harmonizing character, with ability of tuning to a specific person or place. - **Dalai Lama XIV**

A mandala, like any symbol, can be viewed from several aspects: as a structure, as energy, as historical heritage, as a reflection of the collective unconsciousness of people, as traditions, etc. In this chapter, I will describe the main aspects of each of these approaches and try to bring them together into a comprehensive view about the mandala as a resource practice. From a physical point of view, a symbol having a three-dimensional structure (made of metal, stone, wood or any other material) is an oscillatory circuit having its own resonant frequencies (Chapter 1). Moreover, it has been noticed that some volumetric contours have the ability to accumulate ener-gy. The remarkable examples are the pyramids, which have certain proportions as well as hemispheres. This is reflected in the sacred architecture of the temple structures of all religions in the world **(Illus. 1)**. The same effect can be observed in the case of a mandala made in volume and resembling a pyramid (with the central part as the highest point and the outer contour as the base). Based on these observations, the mandala is called the resonator. The physical def-inition of the resonator is as follows: it is an oscillatory system in which oscillation energy is accumulated due to the resonance with a driving force. Typically, resonators have a discrete set of resonant frequencies. In simple terms, this means that the mandala is a kind of energy storage unit for a certain quality. These qualities depend on the structure of the mandala, particularly on its components. In order not to further confuse the concept of the mandala as such and the elements that supplement it, it is worthwhile to turn to the classical definition of the mandala - as the concept of a circle, or rather, a sphere containing a center and borders **(Illus. 2)**.

That is how our ancestors imagined the Universe in a symbolic form. This seemingly primitive vision has the deepest meaning. As it is known, a child is born in the world without self-identification. It is connected with mother in a single whole, and mother in this case acts as a Force replacing the Universe for the child. She feeds and cares, but she also can destroy. Early brain patterns enter our subconscious mind uncontrollably and not critically. In the initial stages of brain formation, the ability to critically evaluate information is absent, and neural networks are not formed yet. Therefore, premature motifs significantly affect our further development. There are a number of theories which suggest that these very early life experiences determine the course of our future life (Grof's theory of perinatal development, etc.). Importantly, as a person grows up and separates from his mother, the subconscious mind automatically puts the person at the center of the mandala, associating with the central force as if it was part of the person and he "owns" it. For example, looking at a watch (which is also a mandala), we understand not only what time it is, but also perceive that time is something that we HAVE. Such perception occurs even if we well understand consciously that we never know how much time we actually have in life, and it is definitely not in our power to own it. There is another subconscious feature of the perception of the mandala, coming from childhood, which plays a significant role in the mandala therapy. Namely, a child who is at the center of attention of his mother and is, thus, connected with power, leading him to feel in balance and safety. The balance here is understood as "everything is fine in my world". That is why, by drawing own mandalas, or working with already created one, a person gains the lost balance and inner support. This is especially important during those times when events or psychological injuries happen in life that knock out the earth under the legs. The first stage of the fight against such significant shocks consists of just centering and gaining at least some kind of internal balance.

Overall, the three main subconscious tendencies that turn on during the perception of the mandala are: **1) to put ourselves in the center, 2) to associate ourselves with the central force and 3) to center, lean and balance**.

As the human race grows (or as the child grows up, if we take it in the context of one human life), the mandala, from a pure matrix with a center and borders, gradually begins to fill up with details. "Others" begin to enter the world of personality. On petroglyphs that have survived to this day, we see mandalas containing images and symbols of seasonal agricultural work, hunting and fishing. The Central Force also takes on several forms: Sun, Water, Fire, Sky and Earth **(Illus. 3)**. The periphery of the mandala is filled with what makes up the human world, the fullness of one's life.

Interestingly, Native American mandalas have one very characteristic feature: their outer edge remains open **(Illus. 4)**. The outer edge of the mandala represents the boundaries of the universe, or the boundaries of the individuality. It also symbolizes the borders of the human life. Thus, it is interesting that for the culture of the American Indians, which has practically everyone seen as a shaman, the concept of borders has clearly a significantly different interpretation. For a shaman, the Life is a vital union with Nature, so close that the grass, streams and trees have their own will and power, just as the human himself is a part of the large natural processes which he is not able to influence. The lack of boundaries for the psyche of a modern man is, frankly, destructive, as the zones of influence and responsibility require a built-in framework. Moreover, the concepts of morality, law and all manifestations of society allowing people to live together do not function effectively in the situation of open borders. Perhaps, that is the reason a real shaman is always alone.

The multilevel mandalas given to us by the Egyptian culture are very thought-provoking **(Illus. 5)**. For the Egyptians, as we know, the animals possessed magical and divine powers. The pantheon of Egyptian gods almost entirely consisted of gods, in a human body, but with the head of a falcon (God Horus), lioness (Goddess Sekhmet), scarab beetle (God Khepri) and jackal (God Anubis). The entire divine pantheon was perfectly structured, where each deity was assigned its own role and task. All of this was very clearly reflected in the mandalas of the ancient times that have come down to us. By the way, the same clear-cut multilevel features also characterize the mandalas of another slave-owning civilization - Mexican Aztecs **(Illus. 6)**. It should be noted that, in comparison with the American Indian mandalas, which also reflect the divinity of natural manifestations, the structure of Egyptian and Mexican mandalas has almost no wavy and irregular lines inherent in the manifestation of emotions. The Egyptian mandalas are an example of clarity and rationality. The same feature is essential in the Jewish and Scandinavian mandalas, along with Arabic, Persian and Tibetan (partially) mandalas **(Illus. 7 and 8)**. This suggests that, in these countries, the knowledge of the world was conducted more through the mind than through the sensually emotional perceptions. Further, in the Jewish and Scandinavian mandalas, the central symbol fills almost the entire inner space, which testifies the feeling of selectivity and deep religious dedication of the people, however, the Arabic and Persian mandalas seem at a first glance the exact opposite: small elements fill the entire space of the mandala in a strictly established order. This reflects the peculiarity of adhering to the strict rules and traditions that personified the Force, which also occupies the entire living space.

The mandalas of the Australian mainland are very consonant with the Charoque Indian mandalas **(Illus. 9)**. They have a lot of natural motives and almost never have clear boundaries. Interestingly, the people have not always been in the center of the universe. Rather, it would be more correct to say that the person has been depicted to not always associate with the central power. Perhaps, the human body was perceived by the aborigines of Australia as something temporary in the life of the spirit. In any case, the harsh climate of the continent, constant fires, droughts and rainy seasons create an atmosphere where a person can die at any time. The state of total physical insecurity is eloquently reflected in the structures of the mandalas.

Tibetan mandalas are the Buddhist mandalas and mandalas of the Bon culture (the original or native culture of Tibet) **(Illus. 10)**. The variety of forms and structures is endless. The mandalas represent the classic "Buddha House", and many of these have been dedicated to the sacred and cosmogonic attributes (Vajrayogini and Lotus mandalas). The mandalas in Tibet are used both as a donation to the Gods and as an instrument of dedication (as an independent spiritual practice). We have learned a lot about the Tibetan "cult" of mandalas after it was allowed to reveal the hidden knowledge to the general public. The travelling Tibetan monks have made the practice of creating sand mandalas and scattering them downwind available in its original form, which is without a doubt very valuable. The structure of the Tibetan mandalas remains classical: in the center is the divinity to which the mandala is dedicated, and the periphery is filled in accordance with the context of life, with the outer edge of the mandala serving as a border that is almost always closed (with the exception of the very ancient mandalas of the Bon tradition, where the God or Demon is shown holding a mandala in the hands). In essence, the root religion of Tibet Bon-Ra has a lot of elements of shamanism, which is reflected in the structure of the mandalas.

Obviously, this brief overview of the mandalas worldwide will not be complete without the mandalas characteristic of India and the Slavic region **(Illus. 11-14)**. These mandalas have a lot in common. The main elements of the ancient Indian mandalas are the floral patterns. Specifically, the yantras **(Illus. 11)** have clear geometric shapes, where the term yantra has been derived from the root yantr (Skt. यन्त्र), meaning "to limit or curb" and belongs more or less to modern Hinduism. Any religious system is guided by the technique of limitation and sin, to keep the people within a framework. The Indian mandalas created during the Vedic period (3300-2800 BC) were characterized by floral-air forms, with many round shapes. The Slavic mandalas of the most ancient Cucuteni-Trypillia culture (c. 5500 to 2750 BC) identified to date consisted very often of a large number of concentric circles combined into complex patterns **(Illus. 12)**. Such structures themselves are remarkable. On the one hand, they are well designed and have clear boundaries, which indicates a highly developed intellect, whereas on the other hand, the circle is an embodiment of the feminine rather than the male principle. This proposes that our ancestors were more likely to have female-mixed expressions of power (which is often the case with nations that did not participate in constant wars). It should be noted that, in India, the style of the soft forms in the mandalas is still preserved and is represented in the practice of Rangoli **(Illus. 13)**. Rangoli is an art form, in which the patterns are created on the floor or the ground using materials such as colored rice, dry flour, colored sand or flower petals. It is usually made during Diwali, Onam, Pongal and other Hindu festivals. The designs are passed from one generation to the next, keeping both the art form and the tradition alive. In contrast, in later times, the features of the Slavic mandalas have been almost lost. The later features contain clear and sharp shapes, based on the sacred geometric patterns **(Illus. 14)**.

I would like to mention that only general trends in the construction and development of mandalas have been described here. Practically, in every nation, one can find exceptions to these trends due to the wide variety of perceptions of Power and related cultural characteristics. Nevertheless, we can see that the times, cultures and religions have succeeded each other, however, the peculiarity of the human subconscious to give the mandala certain functions and properties remained unchanged. The human subconscious refers to the mandalas as a symbol of the interaction of man and the Force and aims to identify itself with It, along with creating its own boundaries and entering a personal life in the mandalas. We perceive the mandalas not only as a phenomenon that exists here and now, but also feel the influence of the centuries-old collective subconscious hidden in it. This information affects us, bypassing the critical perception inherent in the mind as well as avoiding the protective mechanisms and barriers that it creates as a defense against traumatic experiences. Due to this, the mandala therapy can be considered as a resource method. As is known from the classical psychology, a person refuses to see and take a resource precisely because he associates it with some kind of early trauma. For example, a child having seen how his father was cruel to his mother forms a number of painful associations: "relationships are pain", "violence is the only way to communicate", "if you want to survive, obey", etc. Growing up, such a person will be afraid of relationships. It may take years of therapy to change his picture of the world. Working with a mandala that carries a healthy view of the world, the subconscious of such a person can gradually be rebuilt to shift the point of attention from the past traumatic experiences to the present moment. His world will begin to change positively as he begins to manifest himself in a different and more adequate way.

***Image Sources**: Illustrations were partially taken from sites https://www.pexels.com/ and https://pxhere.com/ (Creative Commons Zero (CC0) license).*

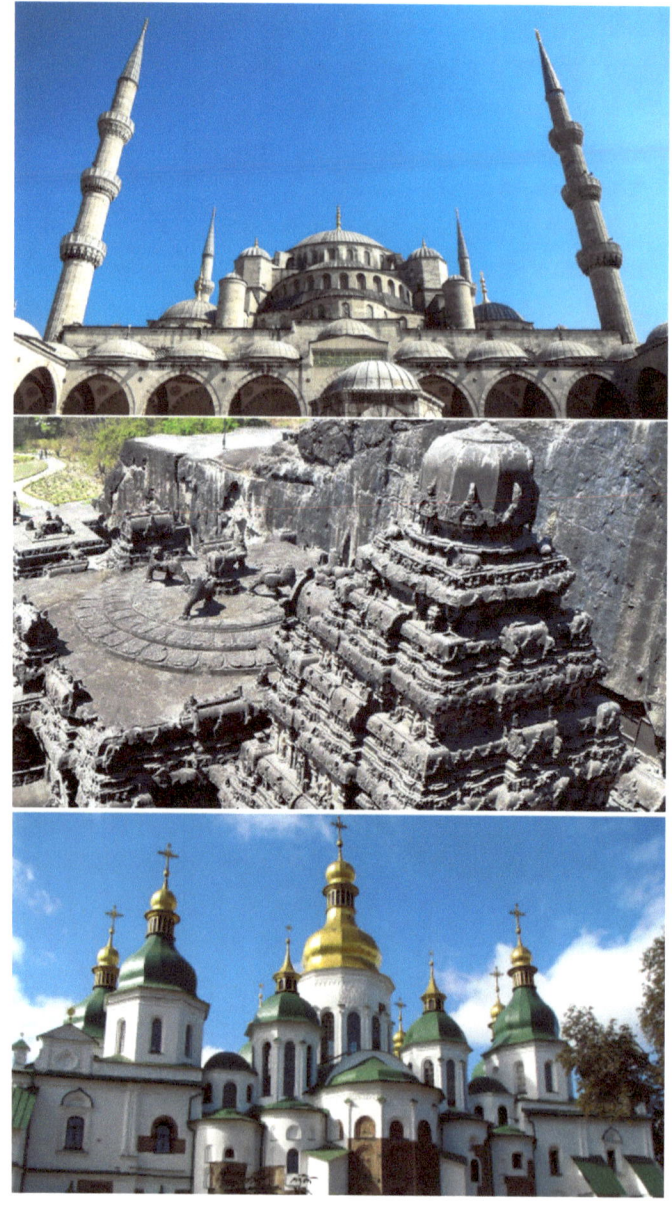

Illustration 1. Sultan Ahmed Mosque, Istanbul, Turkey *(top picture); The **Kailasha** or **Kailashanatha** temple is the largest of the rock cut Hindu temples at Ellora Caves, Maharashtra, India (middle picture); and **Saint Sophia Cathedral** in Kiev, Ukraine (bottom picture).*

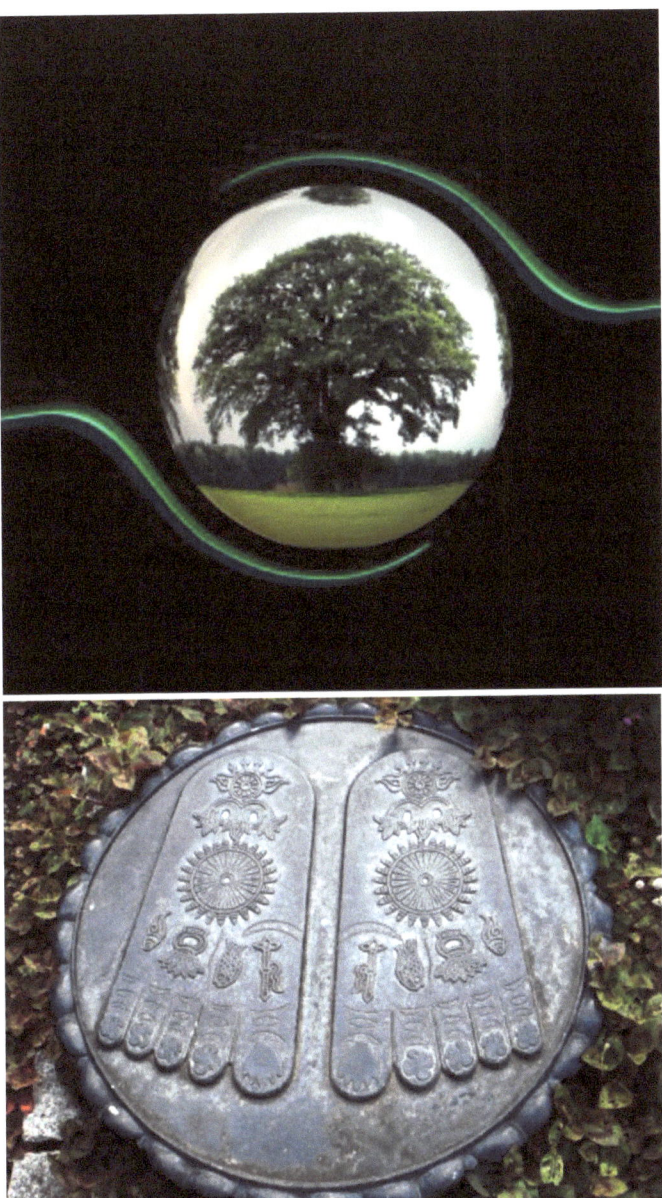

Illustration 2. *The symbolic representation of the mandala - as the Universe and Human Life in the form of a sphere. In the top image, a person places the Life-giving force in the center and subconsciously connects to it.*

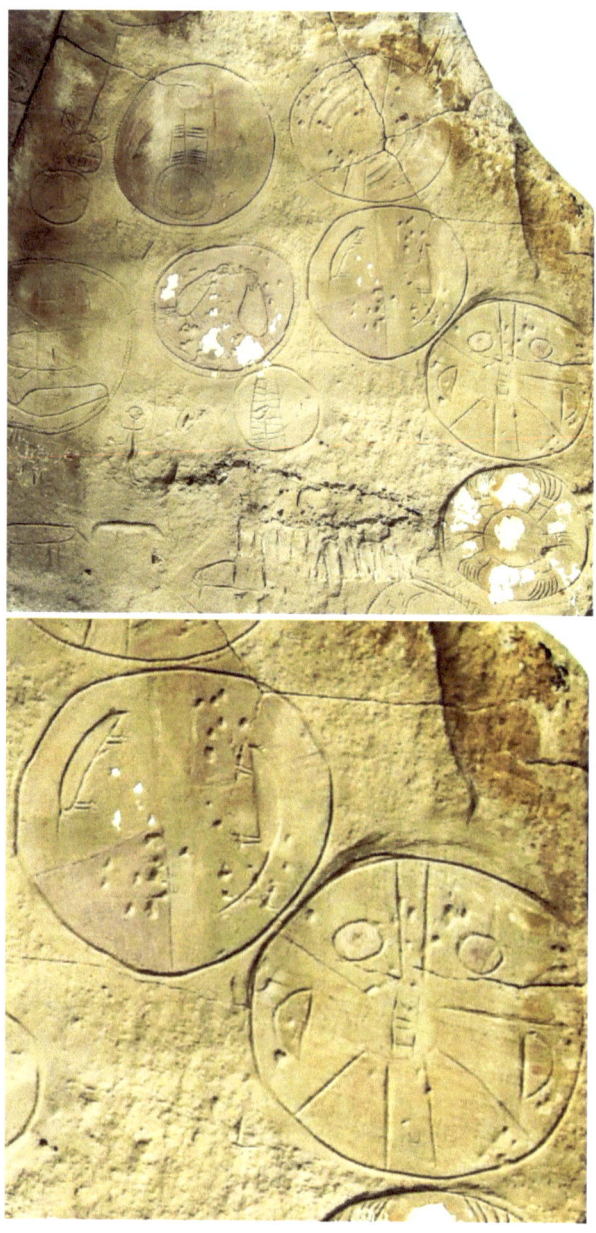

Illustration 3. *Petroglyphs of the American Indians at the Wyoming desert, USA.*

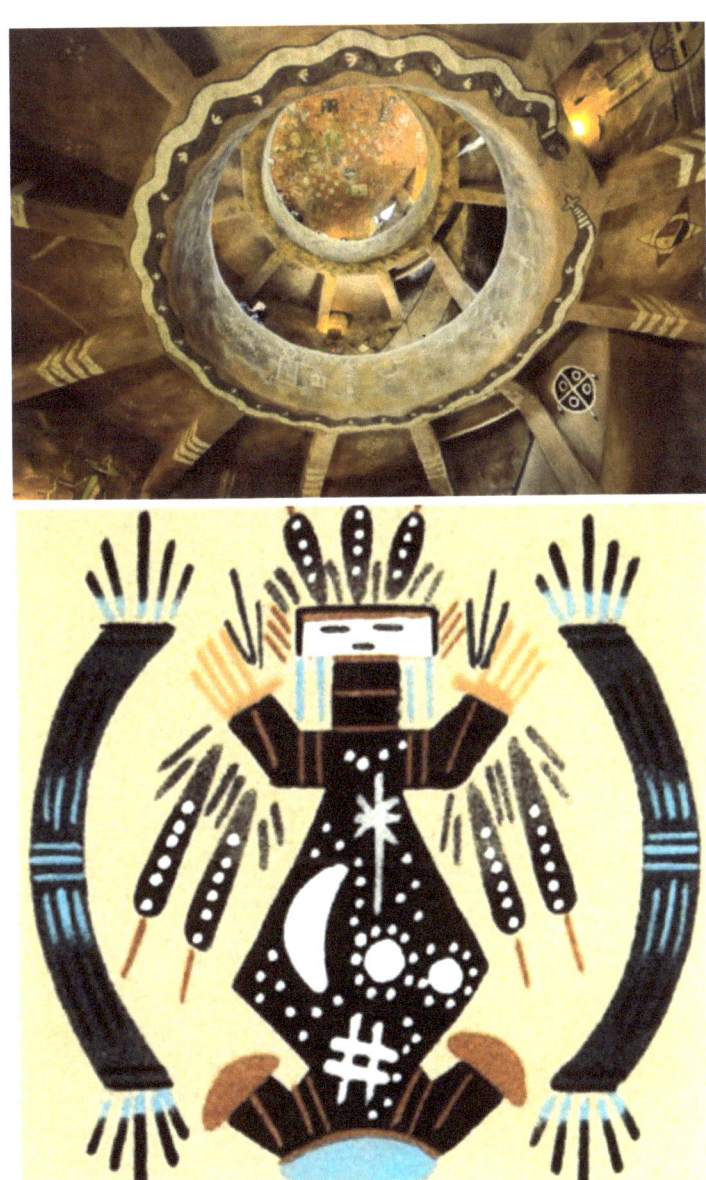

Illustration 4. *The Desert View Watchtower in Grand Canyon National Park, USA. The design is based on the prehistoric architecture in Mesa Verde, Hovenweep, Chaco and Wupatki (top picture); and healing sand mandala "Father Sky" demonstrating the Navajo Indians tradition (bottom picture).*

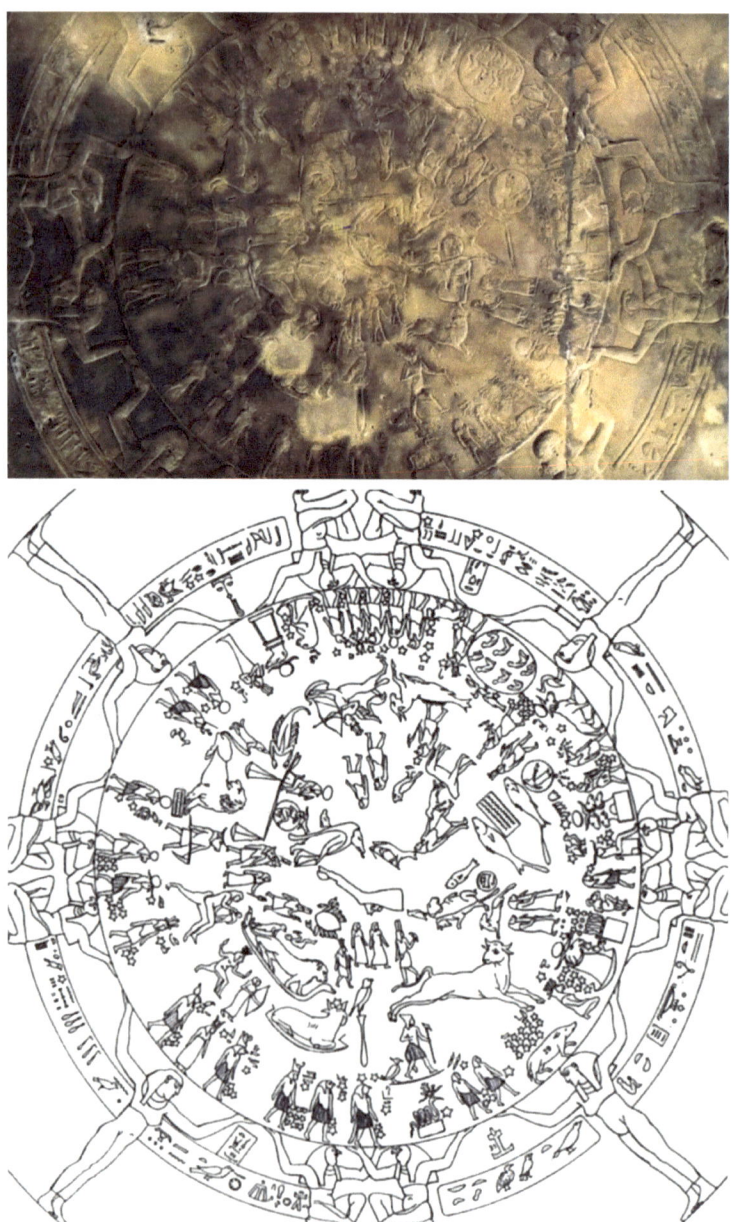

Illustration 5. *The sculptured Dendera zodiac (or Denderah zodiac) from the Dendera Temple complex, Egypt (top picture); and a sketch of Dendera zodiac (bottom picture).*

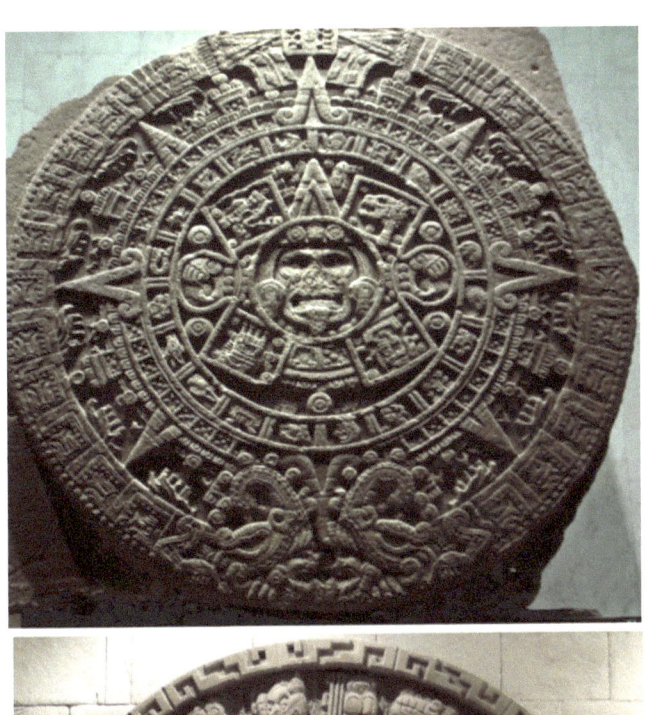

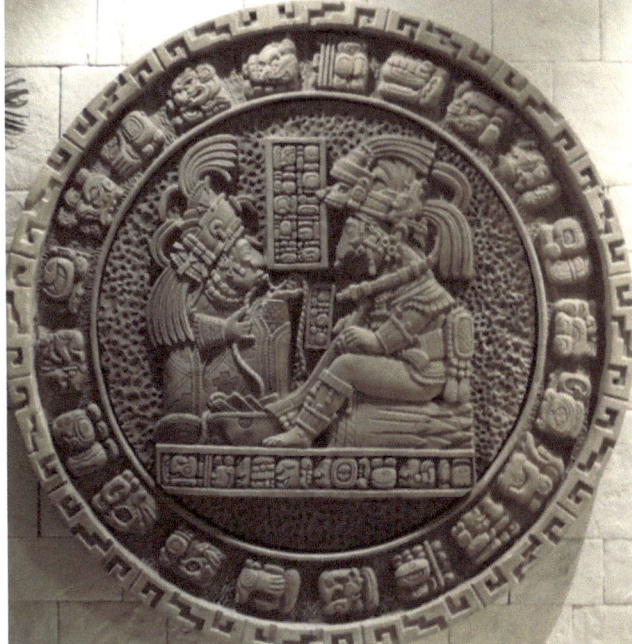

Illustration 6. *The Aztecs mandalas, Mexico: Solar calendar (top picture); and calendar maya (bottom picture).*

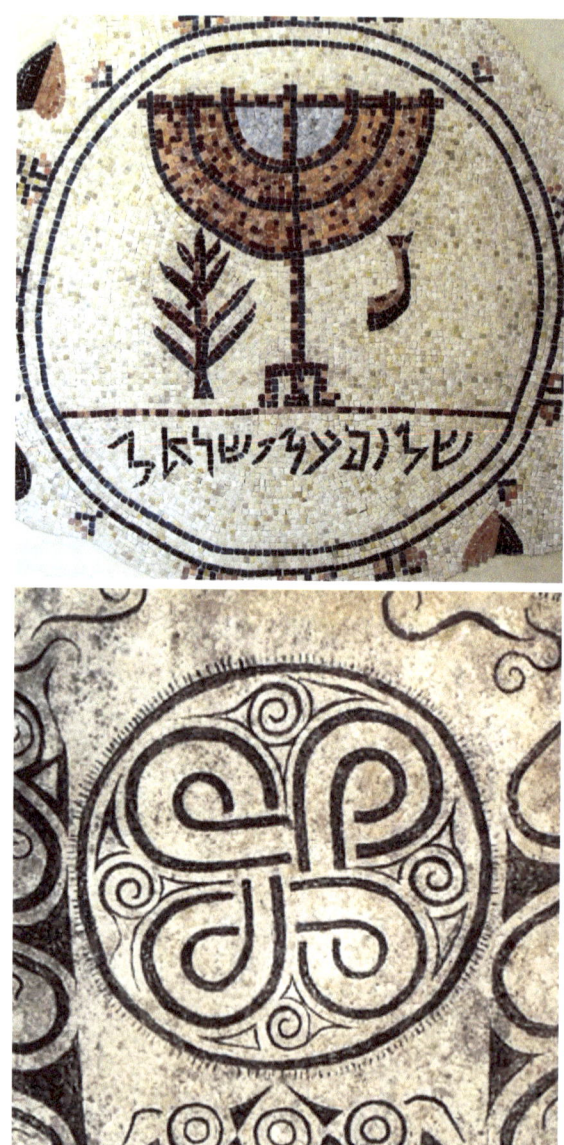

Illustration 7. *Mosaic mandala from the synagogue in Jericho (Tel Sultan) built in the 8ᵗʰ century A.D. (top picture); and looped square migration period picture stone from Havor, Hablingbo, Gotland (1ˢᵗ century A.D.) (bottom picture).*

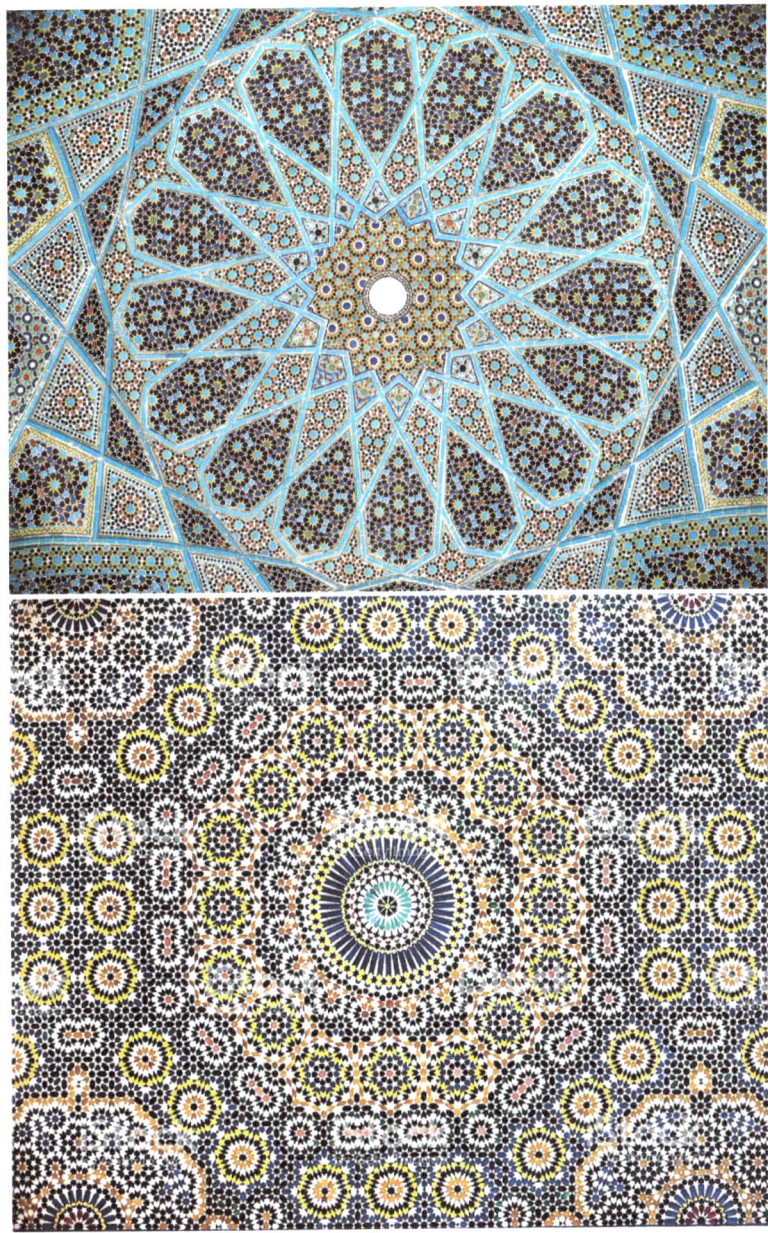

Illustration 8. *Rich mosaic paintings of the mausoleum of Hafez, Shiraz, Iran (top picture); and a traditional Moroccan mosaic pattern tiled wall in the Glaoui kasbah at Telouet, Morocco (bottom picture).*

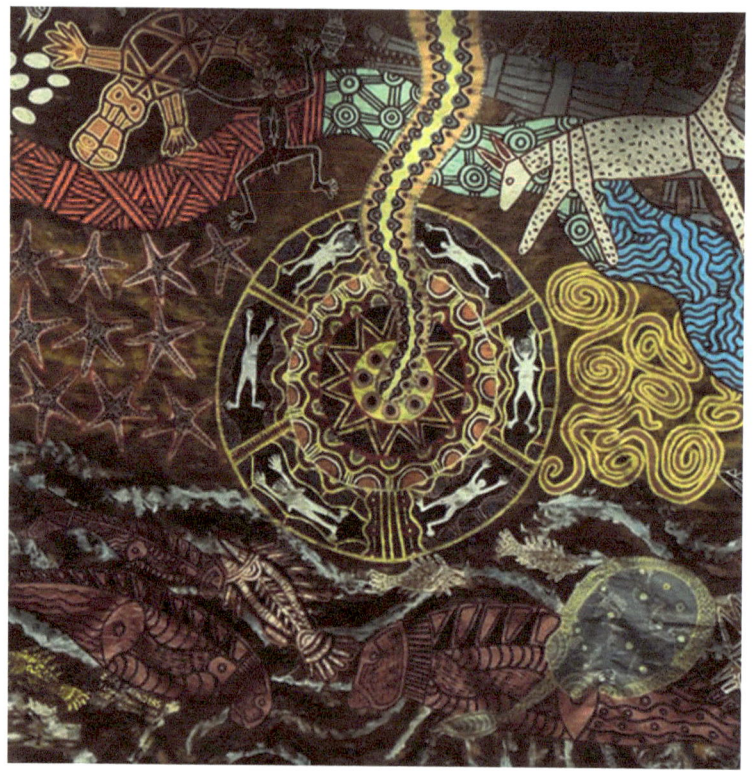

Illustration 9. *The traditional art of the native Australians.*

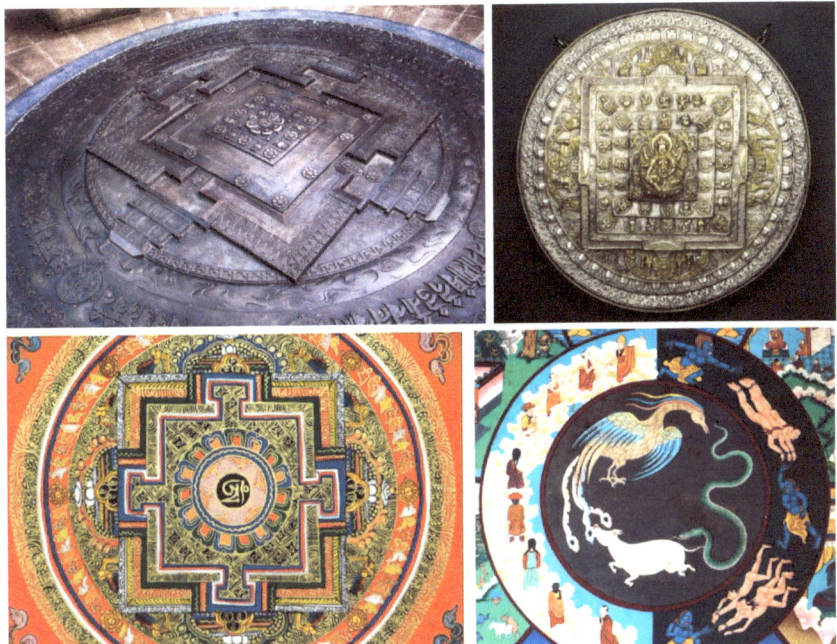

Illustration 10. *Traditional Buddhist Mandalas: Kalachakra (Tibet) (upper left); Tiered Offering Mandala of the Goddess of Wealth Vasudhara (Tibet) (upper right); OM mandala (Nepal) (lower left); and mandala "Wheel of Life" (Nepal) (lower right).*

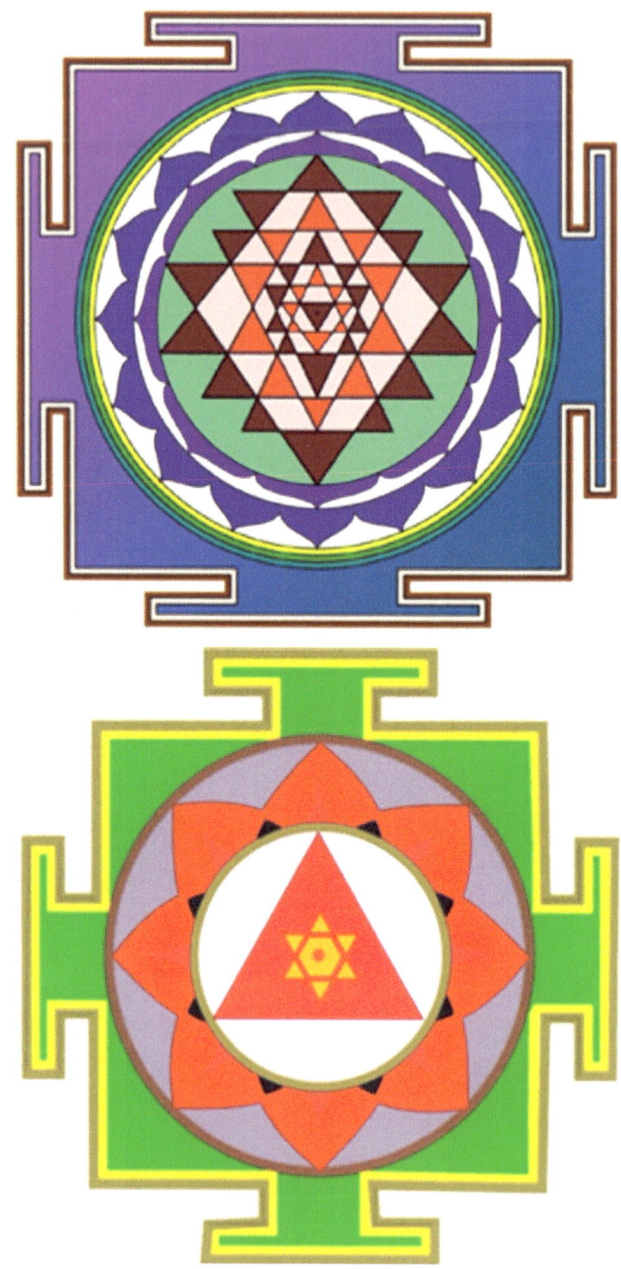

Illustration 11. *Sri Yantra and Yantra dedicated to the God of Wealth Kubera.*

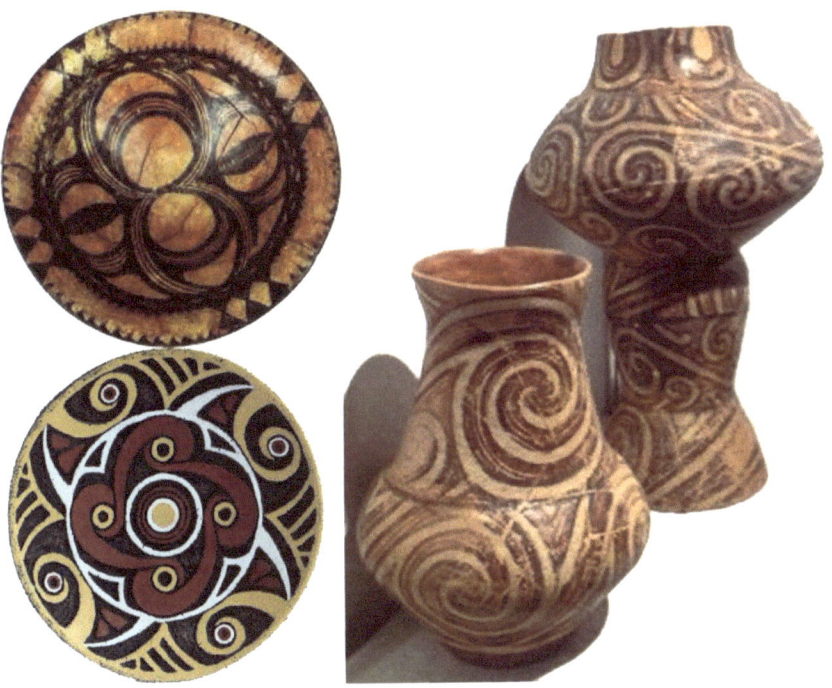

Illustration 12. *Traditional clay pottery of the Cucuteni–Trypillia culture (c. 5500 to 2750 BC).*

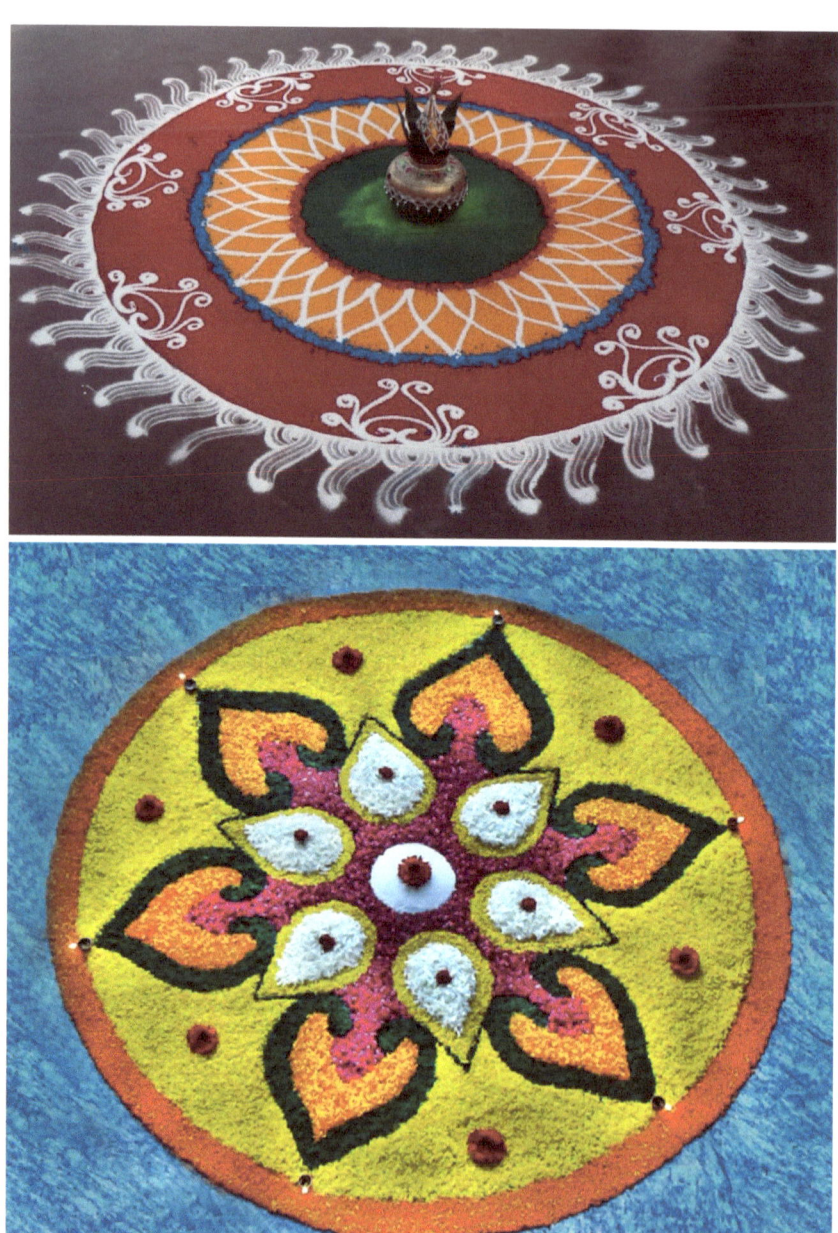

Illustration 13. *Ornamental Rangoli forms, India.*

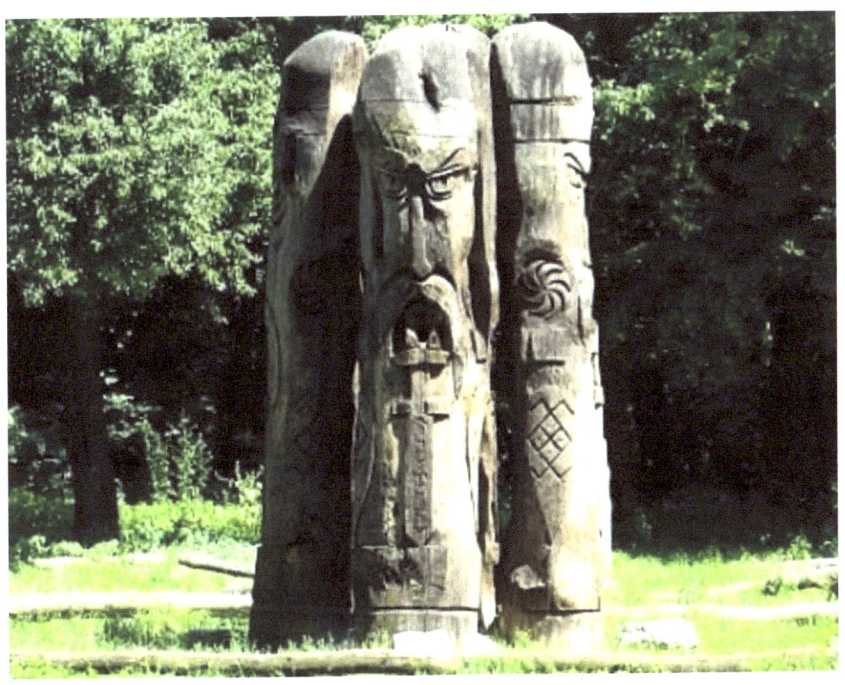

Illustration 14. *Slavic statues of the god Perun with circular symbols in Kiev, Ukraine.*

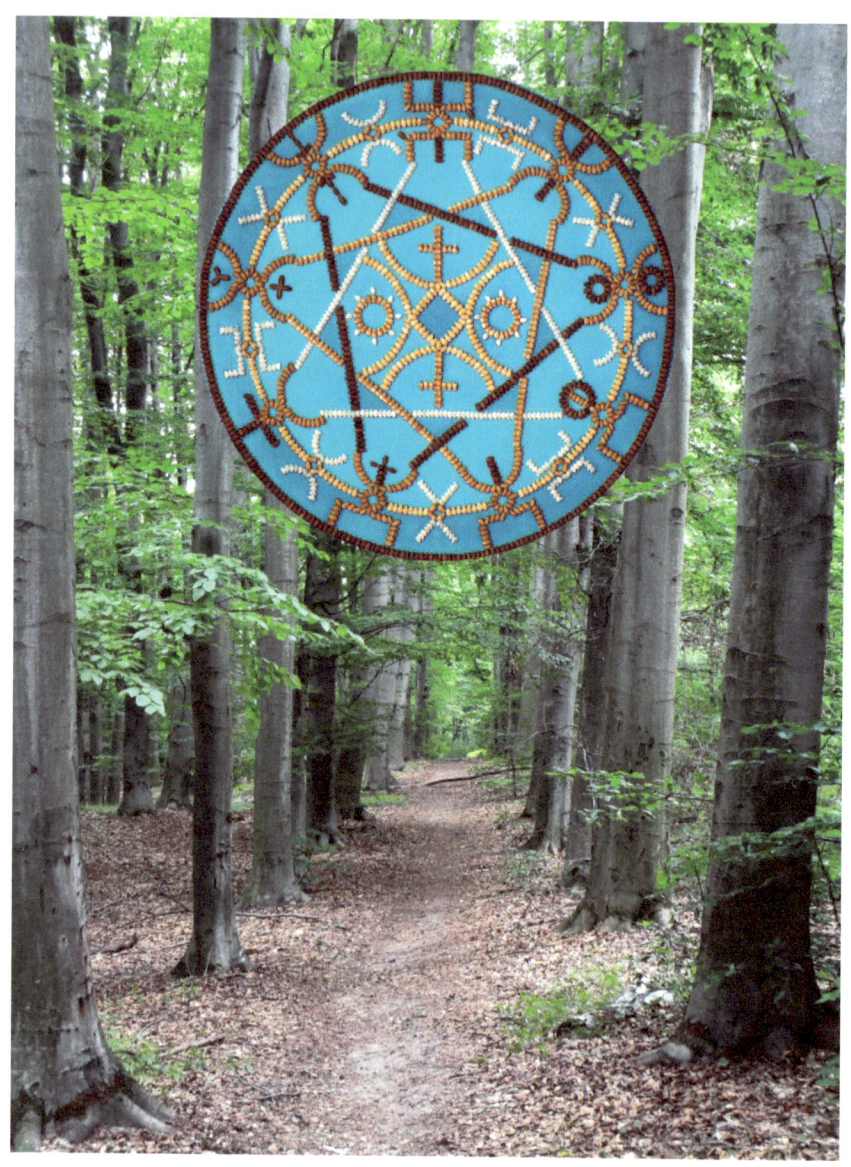

3

Sacred Geometry

When reality reveals secrets, miracles fade away...

There are several approaches to mandala therapy. The first method was invented by Carl Gustav Jung in his own practice of self-knowledge and centering. These days, this approach is often used for therapeutic purposes. Its principle is to create your own daily mandalas, using a basic circle with a center - as an initial template, gradually filled with details. This method not only serves the goal of powerful self-knowledge, but also provides a fairly accurate diagnosis (in the hands of a specialist, of course). It helps to determine the internal psychological state of a person, his problems and limitations. The second method is based on finding a constructive solution to the internal problems of the person, without detailed understanding of the underlying causes of the imbalance (which can take years of therapy). Our internal energy is to some degree reminiscent of a river: if the main waterway is blocked, it will create a bypass. To solve this problem, reference mandalas are used which initially carry the energy of balance, free movement, free growth and a painless transition from one stage of life to another. Such mandalas are created on the basis of structures often called sacred-geometric. The strength here, of course, is not in geometry, as an abstract science, but in the fact that certain geometric patterns are capable of causing in our brain a resonant response characteristic of a particular state. How is this possible? It is easy to recall moments in life when well-chosen music relieves stress, for instance. We hear vibrations, which respond within us, thus, causing resonance in us. The same thing can happen with the right color or smell. It is important to consider that the more individual is the choice of impact or structure (if we return to the mandalas), the higher are the chances of success.

Before listing the basic structures that I most often use in my mandalas, we should understand where they came from. There are a large number of geometric shapes and their combinations, however, several among them stand out that deserve special attention.

At the beginning of the 18th century, the German physicist Ernst Hladni carried out very interesting experiments on the study of sound waves. A metal plate was fixed, sand was poured on it, and a bow was drawn along one of the ribs. The bow created sound vibrations that were displayed on the oscillating plate in the form of structures having a very high level of symmetry **(Illus. 1)**. Dr. Hans Jenny perfected the Hladni experiment. He began to observe interference not only on the plane, but also in the three-dimensional space. To conduct his experiments, he created a special apparatus, termed as tonoscope. He obtained the geometry of the sound vibrations using thin containers filled with various media: sand, wet gypsum and various types of fluids consisting of finely divided media **(Illus. 2)**. While at rest, a suspension of the smallest particles was evenly distributed over the entire volume of the liquid, and the water became turbid. As the container was brought into vibrational motion with different frequencies and amplitudes, the particles in the liquid were folded into ordered and clearly visible geometric patterns with the two-dimensional and three-dimensional structures. Some of the structures very closely resembled the crystalline structures of water (ice) and carbon (the main component of a living organism) **(Illus. 3)**. On the other hand, these same structures have long been used by our ancestors in the construction of mandalas for life (the mandalas that were painted in their dwellings as protective ones). Here are some of them:

Hexagram **(Illus. 4)**: This symbol is present, I am not afraid to say, in every world culture. Among the Slavs, it is the star of Veles, while, it is the star of David among the Jews. In Mesopotamia and the Sumerian tradition, the symbol is assigned to the goddess of fertility and love Ishtar. In India, it is revered as a symbol of the union between Kali and Shiva, considered to be life-saving. In the Buddhist tradition, it is a symbol of Avalokiteshvara. In essence, a symbol is a balancing act of dualities: male and female, internal and external, divine and earthly, material and spiritual, etc. It should be noted that the triangle underlying this structure represents active, fiery and upward-directed energy. Therefore, the symbol is rather actively balancing than passively balanced.

Flower of Life **(Illus. 5)**: The symbol is as ancient as the hexagram. In his works, Leonardo Davinci gave it a special significance. The symbol is displayed on frescoes and bas-reliefs as broadly as a six-pointed star. "The Flower of Life" is the only image that contains every single aspect of creation, all mathematical formulas, every law of physics, every harmony in music and every biological life form", writes Drunvalo Melchizedek in the book "The Ancient Secret of the Flower of Life". Whatever it is, however, the symbol has an almost perfect orderliness and balance. Moreover, this is almost the only symbol with a fractal structure, when each fragment repeats on a reduced scale. In plain language, each part contains complete information about the whole.

Octagram and eight-pointed star **(Illus. 6)**: Despite the fact that the symbols vary in the image, they denote the energy of the Great Mother. The square symbolizes the firmament of earth, and the shape rotated in relation to it by 45 degrees represents the firmament of heaven. Together they serve as a symbol of Alatyr. In the Slavs, this name has several meanings: it is a mythical stone altar that uses the energy of the Mother Earth to materialize the Spirit and anything conceived. Another meaning is "carrying the living soul", i.e, introducing spirituality into the material. The energies of the octagram are considered to be the slowest and most stable on earth.

Nanogram **(Illus. 7)**: This symbol is also called the Star of Iglia. It consists of three triangles and carries a very dynamic structure. The structure is sometimes called the energy of the Primary Fire. This symbol is often used to speed up some processes. It combines very well with the processes related to thinking and superpowers.

Spiral **(Illus. 8)**: It represents another sacred geometric form often used in the construction of mandalas. The spiral is widespread in Nature and is often used in the volumetric execution as a resonator. The shells and our ears are the classic representatives of spirals due to their ability to amplify certain frequencies that are used in the construction of healing structures. Spirals differ based on the direction of flow along them. The clockwise flow is downward, sometimes also called spiritual or masculine, whereas the counterclockwise flow is ascending, earthly and feminine.

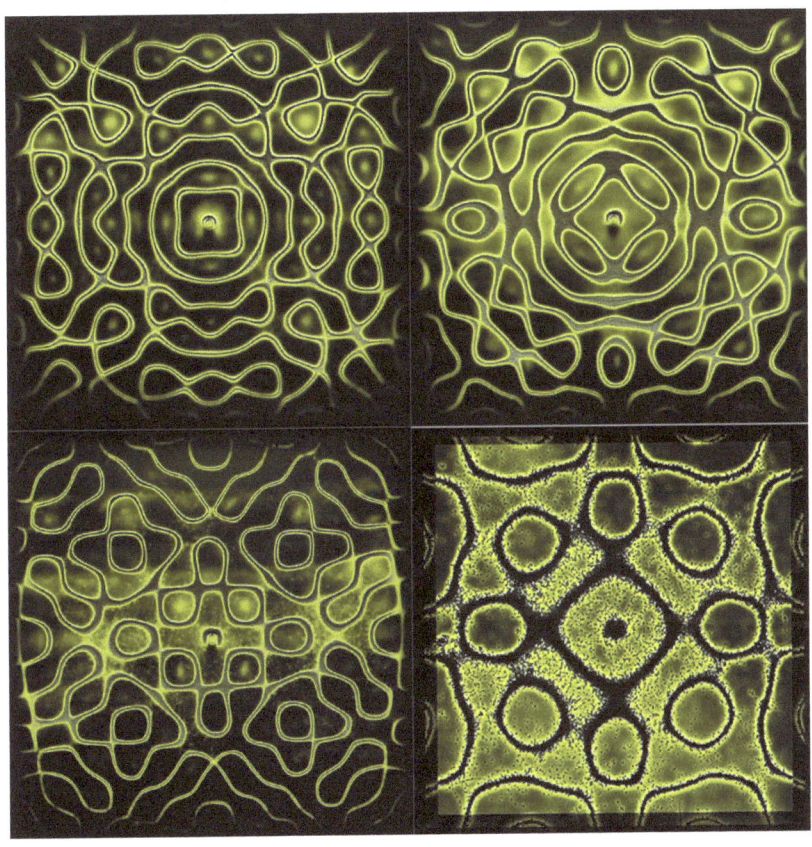

Illustration 1. *Schematic images of the Hladni diagrams.*

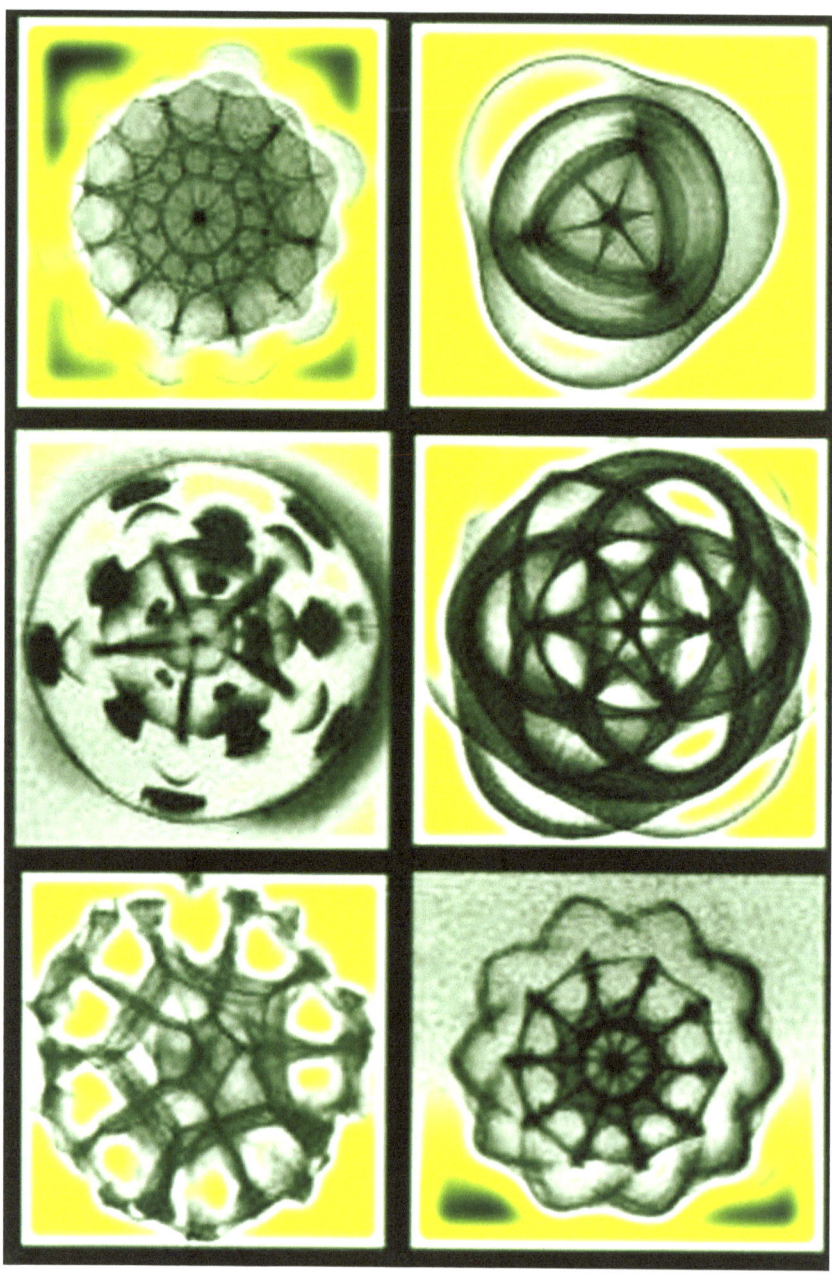

Illustration 2. *Schematic images of the Hans Jenny diagrams.*

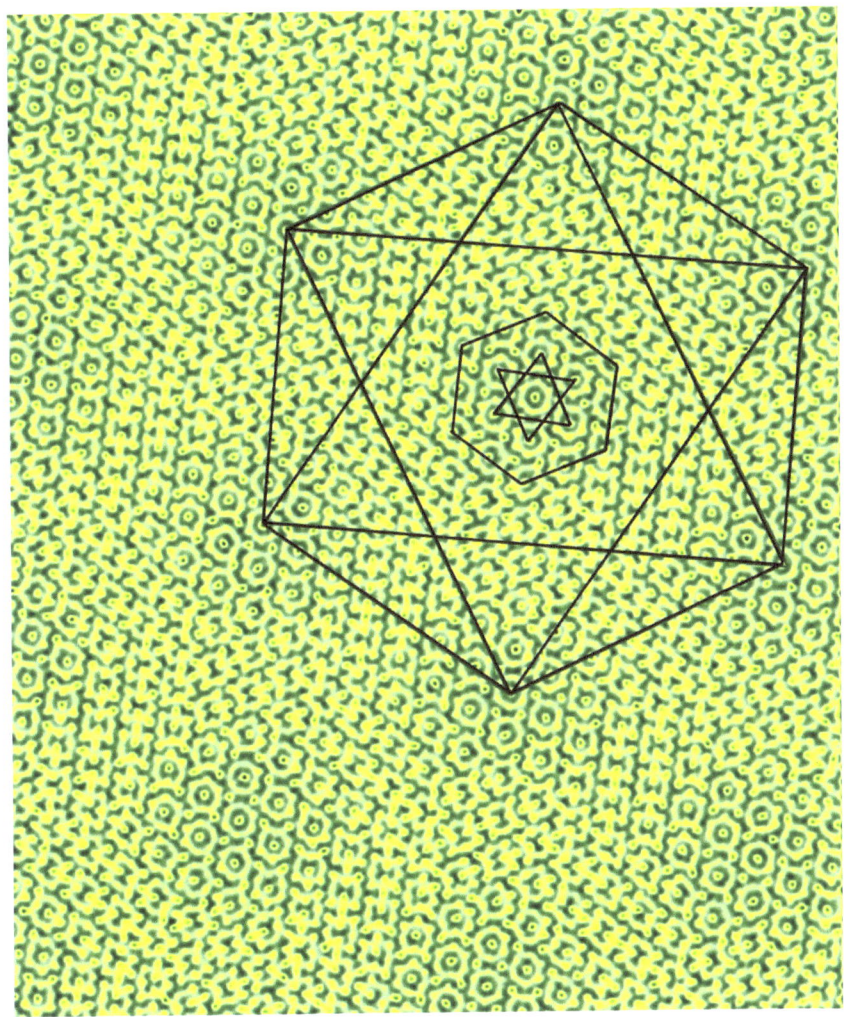

Illustration 3. *Schematic image of the atomic structure of ice.*

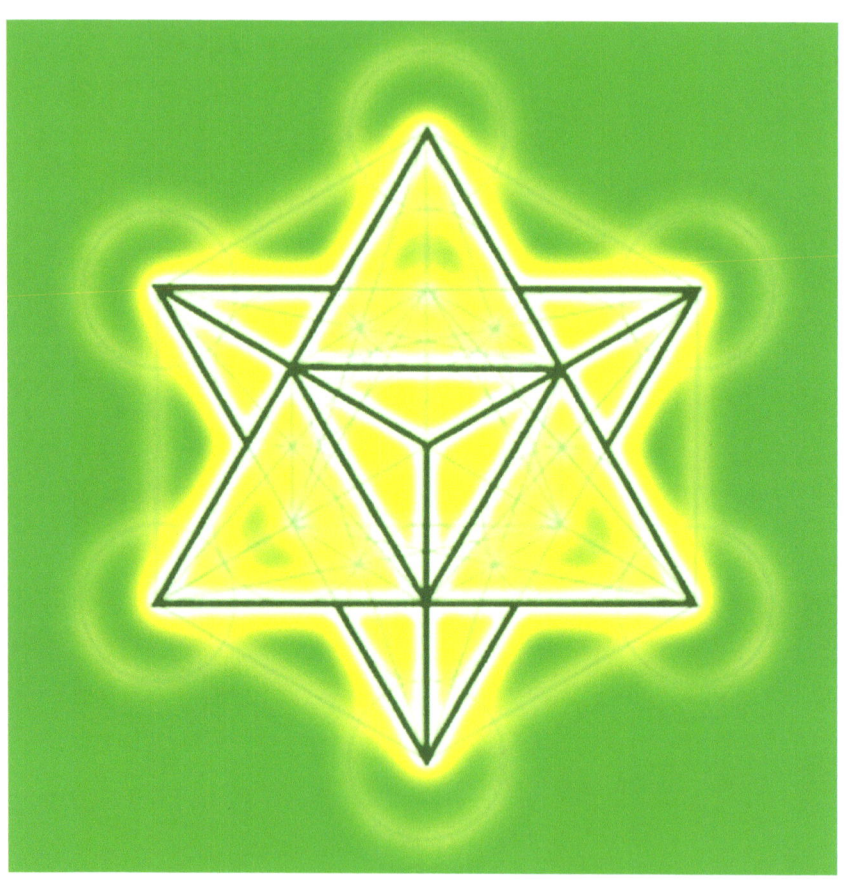

Illustration 4. *Hexagram.*

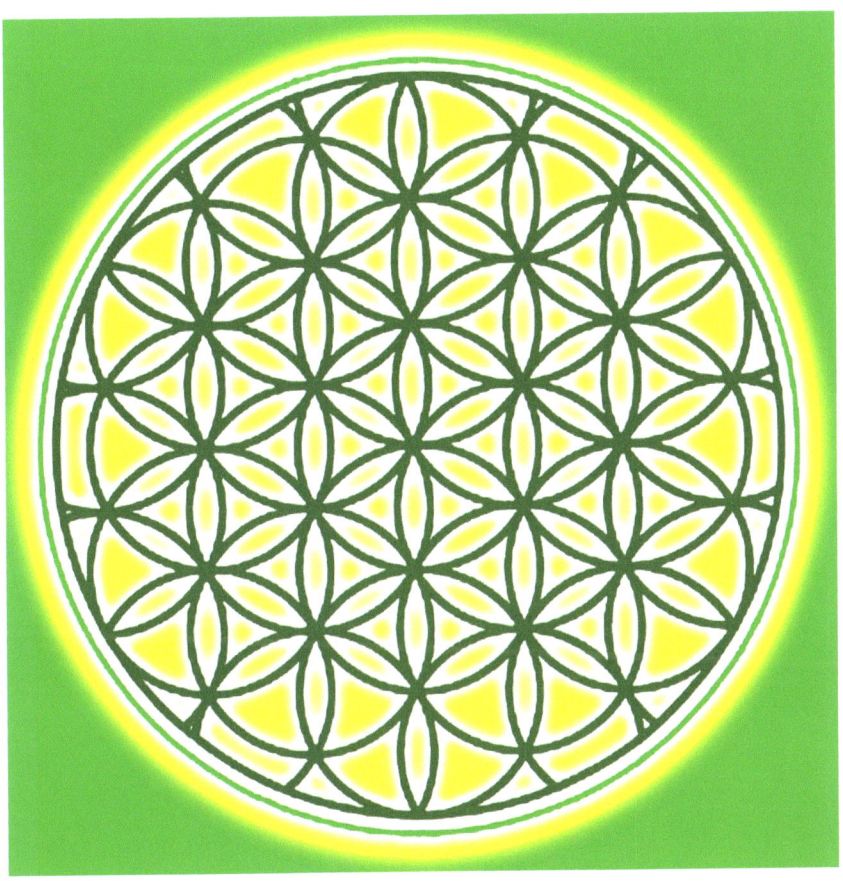

Illustration 5. *Flower of Life.*

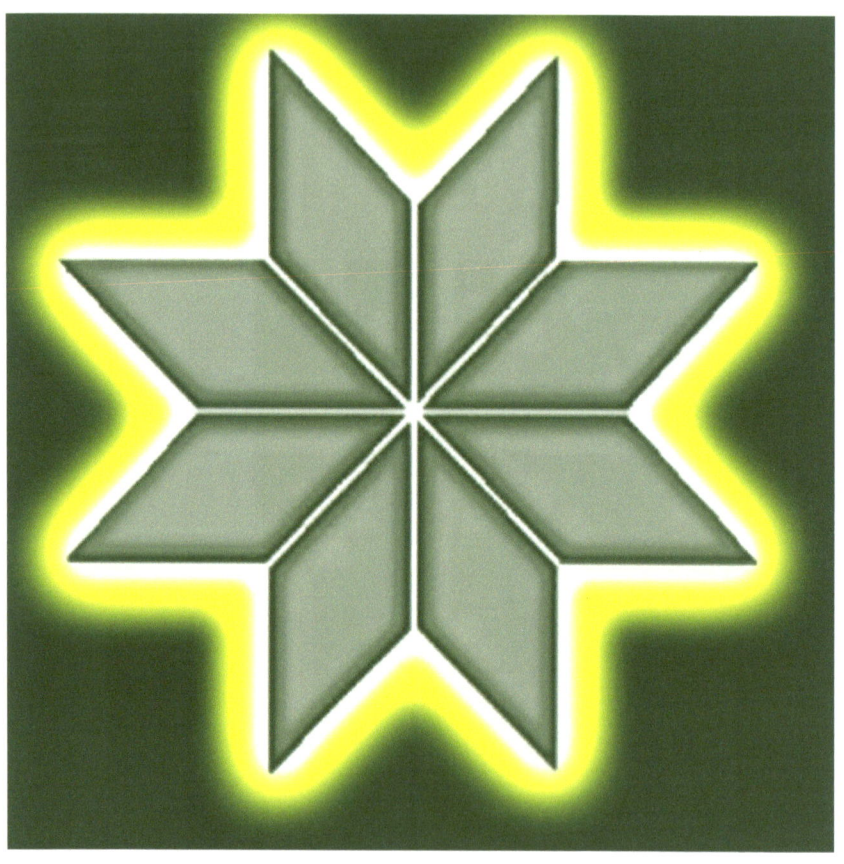

Illustration 6. *Alatyr.*

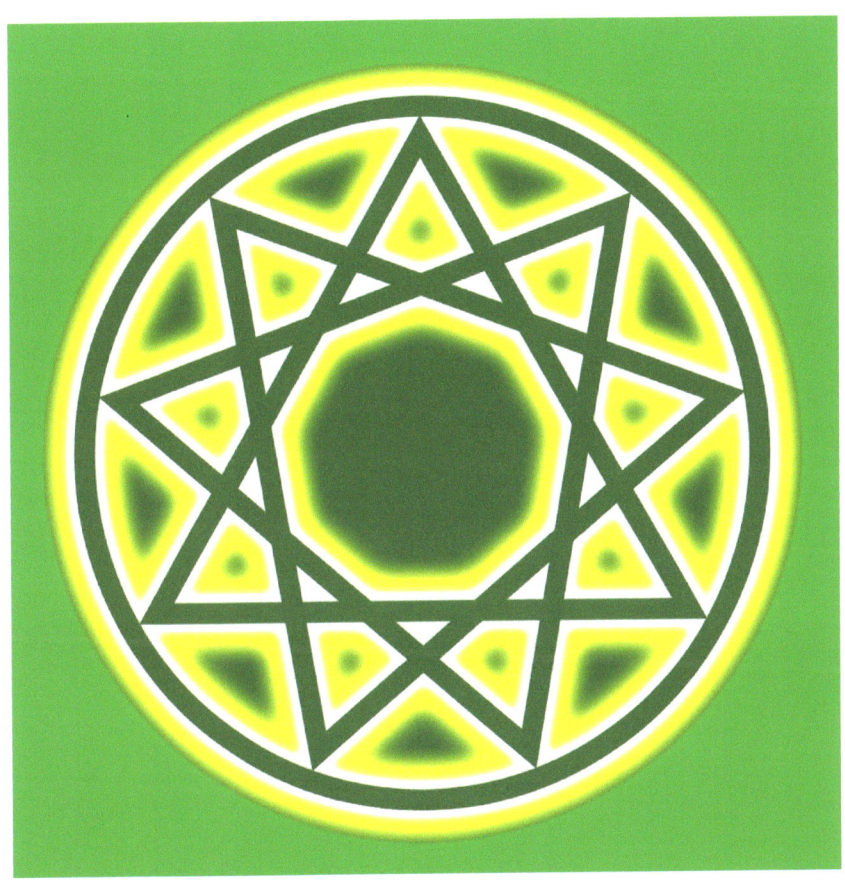

Illustration 7. *The Star of Iglia.*

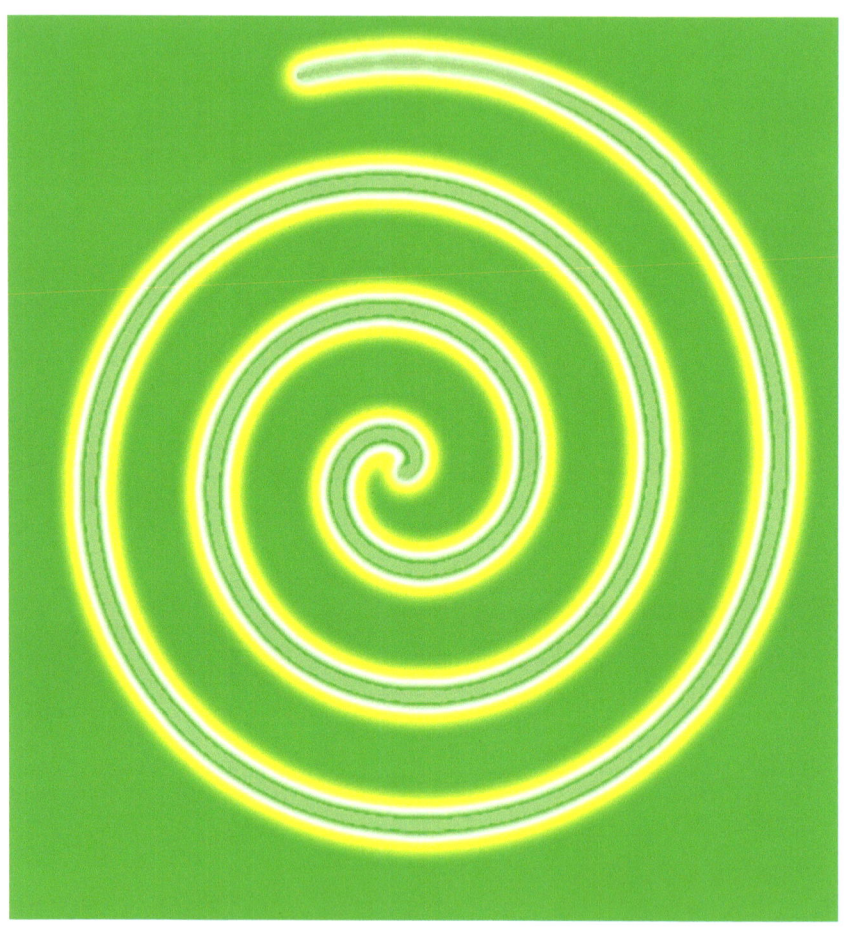

Illustration 8. *Spiral.*

4

Runes

A symbol is "a sign by which a phenomenon is recognized in its deep irrational essence"

The desire for control is one of the dominant features of the human mind of the 21st century. Control and predictability are conditions that create a sense of security in our ever-changing world. However, deep down, we know that control is an illusion same as the most of our ideas about the world order. It is solely due to the global nature of the world order with countless chaotic probabilities that can happen at any moment, which neither statistics nor any of the existing philosophical and religious paradigms can predict. However, as the wise say, in spite of the fact that there is no security in this world, one can still feel safe in it. This is achieved, in most cases, due to simplification. The complex phenomena are gradually simplified to their symbolic representation. For example, in ancient times, a sign of well-being was the presence of food and implements that help to constantly renew this food. Over time, people invented the monetary system where the well-being was not calculated in kilograms of mammoth meat stored in the caves, but in terms of the amount of gold and silver coins as well as precious stones. Later, paper money replaced gold, and. in the modern world, a plastic credit card acts as an image of well-being. Obviously, a piece of plastic is absolutely unsuitable in food, however, it is a symbol of those funds that are in the corresponding bank account, and which can be cashed out with food and other household goods. Symbols, which a person surrounds himself with, create a less predictable and controlled reality.

Each symbol carries a certain information layer, which contains the original phenomenon in all its complexity and versatility. The human brain often lacks the energy resource to perceive the incoming information in its fullness, and it perceives only its "scheme", in the form of a symbol, despite the fact that the subconscious, according to neurobiologists and epigenetics, preserves the entire information package as fully as possible. That is why the entry into the subconscious and subsequent influence is carried out through a system of symbols. This system is used by not only professional psychologists, psychiatrists, art therapists, etc., but also people who have power and control, including representatives of all religious doctrines without exception. It should be noted that in countries where the connection with ethnic roots is still alive, the ability to properly direct people consciousness with the help of symbolism is still actively used to this day. For instance, folk patterns are used in dishes, clothes and jewelry.

Let's get back to the main topic of this chapter, namely runes. There are many runic ranks belonging to the different ethnic cultures. What they have in common is that each system of runic symbols claims not only a holistic description of the laws of the universe, but also a complete set of the standard natural and social energies that can be touched using runes as a kind of resonators of these energies. Simply, the interaction with the rune allows you to open and feel those emotions and sensations that are characteristic of the energy designated by it. The examples include rune Love (a feeling that broadens the heart and creates deep agreement with everything that happens around), rune Prosperity (a feeling of fullness and abundance), rune Security (a sense of security and support), etc. If you believe Karl Gustav Jung, both the ancient symbols themselves and their deepest meaning are embedded in the brain of every person as a result of the collective unconscious or evolution. Therefore, a conscious concentration or contemplation of sacred forms automatically immerses the brain in those phenomena described by the symbols. For example, concentration on the symbol of Growth automatically triggers internal mechanisms of development at all levels: physical, spiritual, mental, etc.

The main difficulty is that very rarely a person is able to hear his response to a particular runic symbol. Usually, this is gained by the practice of listening to oneself and one's body reactions. The situation is somewhat akin to a musician who, when looking at a sheet of music, is able to hear it. More often, we have to deal with the situation described in the classic film "Groundhog Day": "Do you see a groundhog? Not? But he is!" In the runic practice, there are always two principles - the rune, which has its own individual energy, and the person, who captures this energy, interacts with it and directs it in the desired direction. As there are no two completely identical people, there is no general unified theory about the outcomes. Everyone receives and experiences the information at their own level, and this level tends to change over time. In this chapter, I want to share exactly my vision, in no way claiming the ultimate truth. Each sign from the rune row (I mean Alatyr runes) is a symbol of some natural principle, which in one way or another interacts with a person in the process of his life: path, fire, growth, love, balance, etc. So, in Alatyr runes, three pronounced levels are visible. The upper level (open upward arc, square, triangle, etc.) symbolizes the inner world of a person, his soul and connection with the higher worlds. The middle level (central rhombus) symbolizes the transition from the spiritual to the material world, while the lower level (open downward arc, square, triangle, etc.) symbolizes the real material world. The runes I use in practice are briefly described in the following.

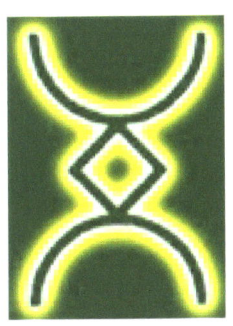

1. Rune Path (The Road)

Rune Path carries the energy of movement into life. The movement here is an antagonist of stagnation. It helps to adjust the subconscious mind, "there is always a way out, even if you don't see it right now". Or, as the wise say, "do it to understand". Very often it helps to get rid of fears along the way, otherwise, a person may motionlessly wait for a "good moment" for years fearing changes. The art of small steps is one of the gifts the rune Path gives to him.

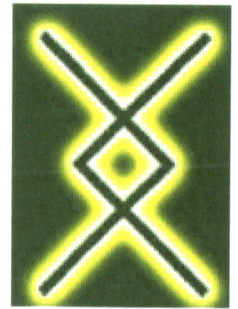

2. Rune Protection (Defense)

It is clearly visible from the shape of the arches of the rune Protection that its main task is to cut off anything unnecessary. A clear movement towards the goal, without spraying energy on the sides (energy saving). Rune Protection is helpful when you need some kind of armor that protects against blows. However, it has to be practiced carefully, as it closes the person from the entrance to the exit. A person practicing with this rune may become insensitive to the subtle external events and people nearby. This rune is the warrior's armor, which is worth removing in peacetime.

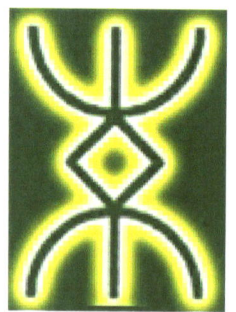

3. Rune Prosperity

It is a rune that sets up a person's subconscious mind in a state of abundance and well-being. Moreover, additional straight lines located in the center of the celestial and earthly arcs indicate that abundance means the realization of talent and innate abilities embedded in each person. I take it from the spiritual world, realize it in my reality, and give it back to the earthly world. It is, thus, the balance between "take" and "give". Practice with this rune helps to free the subconscious from the feeling of a chronic lack of wealth, love, recognition, etc.

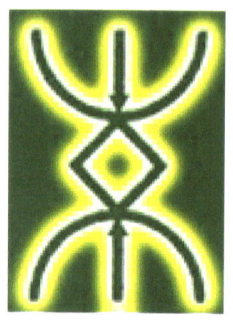

4. Rune Concentration

This rune is invaluable in the cases where we cannot focus our attention on something important and constantly live with the feeling that all life energy is smeared with a thin layer without bringing any positive results. Practice with this rune will be very useful to dreamers who have no hands-on real life. This is the rune of energy concentration in the current moment. It also serves as a wonderful help in subtle practices and work requiring maximum attention.

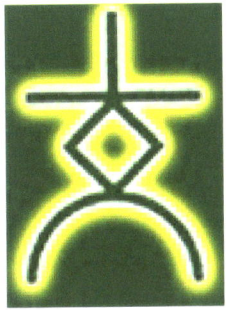

5. Rune Heaviness

In the structure of rune Heaviness, an upper "divine" part is not limited. In figurative language, the firmament of heaven presses on its shoulders and presses it to the Earth. The rune will be extremely useful where a person subconsciously feels his lightness, non-earthing, lack of weight, etc. The person can scream, freak out, lose his temper, however, for others, he simply does not have enough weight. Thus, this rune brings authority and inflexibility.

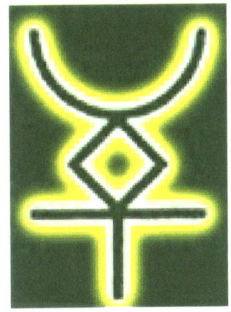

6. Rune Lightness

It is the opposite of the rune Heaviness. The earth's lower structure is open, which creates a feeling of pushing and lightness. This energy is necessary when a person sticks to something. Often this is the result of excess ballast and sometimes even a resource. It is wonderful to practice it in situations where a person is not able to perform an action because of endless reflection on the situation, weighing it on all scales and considering it from all sides. Or, in cases where an infinite number of actions fall on a person at the same time, and instead of raking them one by one, the person falls into a stupor and does nothing at all.

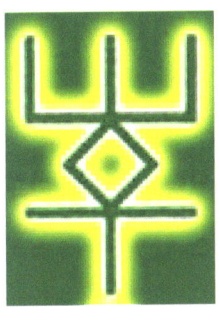

7. Rune Breath

It is one of the cleansing runes. In the upper celestial structure, there is an element symbolizing the flow of energy, which has a set goal (trident). Such energy serves to get rid of all energy blocks along the way. The lower earthly structure symbolizes the unlimited ascending earthly flow that pushes. The rune Breath is good to practice when a person needs the soft unlocking of the movement, an expansion of opportunities, to develop a taste for life, to experience new perspectives, etc. We often say, "get around the problem". For such practices, the practice of rune Breath is highly helpful. It is also the rune of healing the lungs.

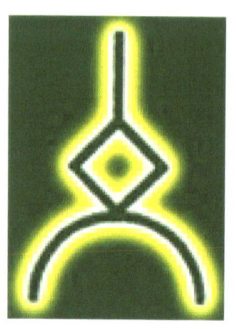

8. Rune Purposefulness

This is the rune representing the formation of a bright strong goal, which can be realized in the earthly world. The rune is very useful for practice in those places, where, due to the complexity or ambiguity of the task, the movement stops without clear understanding where to take the next step. It is a rune of planning and discipline in all fields of life. This rune motivates the prioritization and movement towards the set goal. This is also the rune of powerful will to achieve the unthinkable.

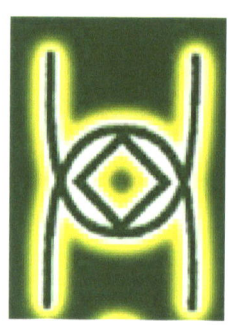

9. Rune Sacrifice (Sign of the Warrior)

The structure of this rune is such that the central square, symbolizing the transition from the spiritual to the material world, is as if in an additional circuit opens up to the spiritual world and down to the earthly world. It represents a world of open opportunities and additional protection for direct interaction with them. Practice with this rune allows you to enter the states of courage and action. In fact, any conscious change in our lives, as well as the realization of the desired, requires these conditions. The way out of the familiar is always scary. It scares even when the person himself is no longer able to endure his usual way. The energy of the first step into the unknown, determination, composure and maximum sensual inclusion are the energies that the Warrior rune carries in itself, thus, immensely benefiting the practitioner.

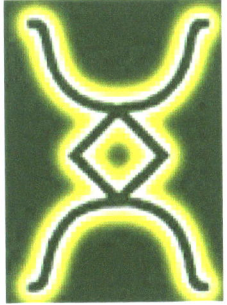

10. Rune Satiety (Fullness)

Practice with this rune awakens the state of fullness in the subconscious. Very often we are unable to stop the temptation, "more, more, it's not enough for me, I am hungry," precisely because of the state of the inner gaping chimney through which our energy flows. Most often, such temptations result from a trauma we may have suffered. For instance, the grandmother may have malnourished during the war, and now we eat both for ourselves and for grandmother! The practice with this rune allows you to close such a funnel. The rune is very effective as an independent subject of practice and combines wonderfully with other energies, for example, runes Love, Prosperity and Power.

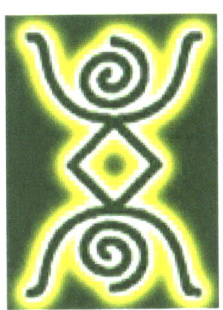

11. Rune Whirlwind

This rune combines the energy of upward and downward energy flows. Practice with this rune carries two main functions: cleansing and balancing. It helps the subconscious to balance the energy flows in the body, while accelerating the state of stagnation. Often the actions after practice with this rune occur very organically and without the strain characteristic of resistance.

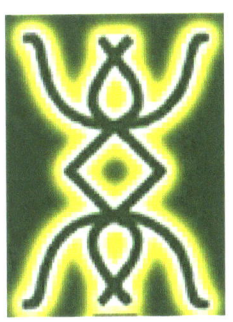

12. Rune Love

The structure of this rune combines the energy of fullness and the energy of the birth of a new life. In fact, this is the energy of the 'continuation of life'. We take energy from the world of the 'spirit' to create a new life in the world of 'matter', and we take energy from the world of 'matter' to create a new life in the world of 'spirit'. Practice with this rune not only expands our energy possibilities for creating a new one, but also heals the body, especially beneficially affecting the heart center. The energies of peace, concord, calm and confidence appear when working with it continuously.

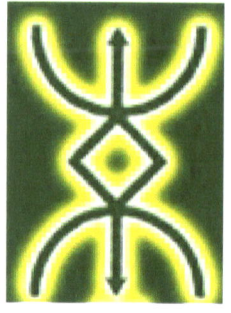

13. Rune Scattering

It is the rune of transformation and protection. Its peculiarity is that it stretches or dissipates the state to which the practitioner is directed. You can work with it to relieve the states of fear, panic or depression. It alleviates all symptoms, transforming the global problems first into local problems and subsequently the transformation of these problems into opportunities. This is also the rune of meditation and rest. It has also healing functions if the task is to remove the excess of something from the body.

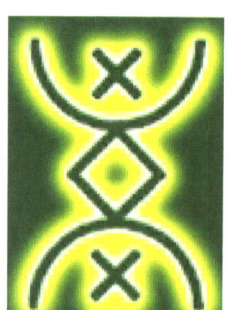

14. Rune Lock

The energy of this rune is protective in nature. It stops the movement. Practice with it can be useful if we feel that the movement in our life is not directed in the desired direction. All kinds of addictions, from work to alcohol, can be alleviated by working with rune Lock. Also, this rune can be used for protection when we feel that the negative energy has been directed at us. With its help, our subconscious mind learns to close its own field from outside influence. It is also the rune of preservation.

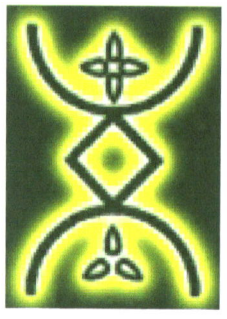

15. Rune Water

The elemental rune, like all elemental energies, has a colossal resource that opens up with prolonged practice. First of all, the rune Water represents purification from misinformation. Thus, it is the rune of information and communication. It is also the rune of diagnosis and intuition. Practice with it allows the ossified structures to become more flexible and fluid. This is especially useful when we mentally rest in a hopeless situation and are not able to see the way out. Practice with it helps to feel the true cause of what is happening and to see something which is hidden in the shade. Care should be exercised while practicing rune Water. If there are significant problems in the subconscious, this element can manifest itself in the most unexpected way.

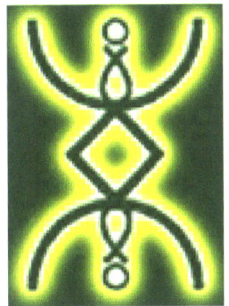

16. Rune "Our Civilization"

This rune allows the understanding and feeling of large processes in large and small manifestations. It is the rune of scientists, analysts, teachers and guides. Practice with it helps to expand the horizons of understanding and cognition. It helps to feel the social trends. It is also the rune of deep meditation. It is also possible to apply it to what practitioners call the "world library" (the information field where all the knowledge of mankind is collected). Carl Gustav Jung called this space the collective unconscious. The rune requires a certain level of self-understanding and ability to work with the unconscious.

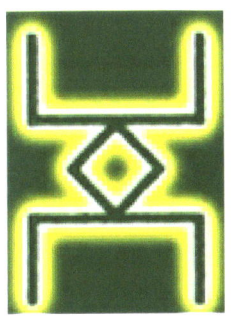

17. Rune Stream

It is one of the most powerful runes of the movement of energy with various properties. This rune is rarely used in practice by itself. More often, it is used in conjunction with runes symbolizing certain energies: wealth, love, healing, etc. Practice with it allows one to form the paths of energy movement and clean them if there is a feeling that the channel is energetically blocked or clogged. Thus, this rune is wonderful to practice when it comes to the energy channels of our body. In classical Tibetan and Chinese medicine as well as acupuncture practices, the human body is pierced by energy channels, leading to the free circulation. The mental movement of the rune along these channels can significantly improve the practitioner's well-being.

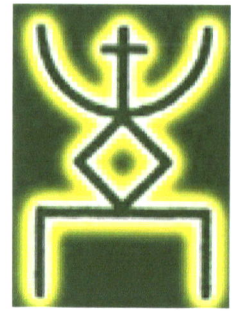

18. Rune Victory

This rune carries the energy of successful completion of projects and undertakings. The structure of this rune is such that it combines the leading spiritual principle "from above" and active targeted energy directed to the material, leading to the earthly realization of this principle "from below". Practice with this rune helps to competently and adequately plan new beginnings and actively implement them. Also, this rune is a healer. Depression, deep disbelief in one's strengths, self-abasement and depreciation can be easily corrected with regular practice. "Happiness is not as blind as it is imagined. Often it is the result of a long series of measures, true and accurate, not seen by the crowd, and preceding the event", said Catherine the Great. Rune Victory helps to build one's behavior and actions so that a successful result of efforts becomes inevitable.

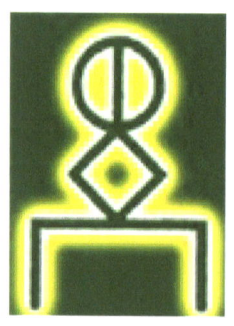

19. Rune Growth

This is the rune of the colossal resource of growth, development and realization, embedded in each of us by Mother Nature. It carries the energy of the natural course of events when one state is replaced by another, thus, forming cycles. These cycles are represented as: the emergence of a new cycle (spring), the accumulation of experience (summer), the harvesting and dumping of waste (autumn), and summing up and preparing for a new cycle (winter). Immobility in one state leads to a halt in the natural process of development, leading to the stagnation of energy. Practice with the rune Growth allows one to move the wheel of the year further and go to the next stage after stagnation. Rune Growth is also a powerful healer of the organs responsible for the birth of a new life.

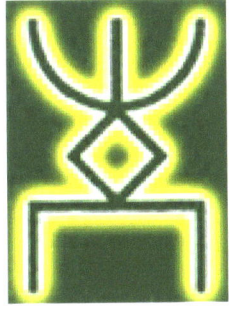

20. Rune Wind

This rune symbolizes one of the most powerful elements - the element of air. It is the rune of intelligence, information and purification. One of the key benefits that comes by practice with this rune is the feeling of freedom and flight, along with the ability to look at the problems superficially, "from top to bottom". After this view, the solution very often becomes apparent even without additional analysis. The rune is also used to clear internal restrictions.

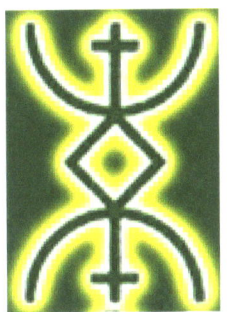

21. Rune Awareness

It is the central rune that helps awaken our sleeping superpowers: clairvoyance, clairaudience, clarity of knowledge and intuition. Practice with this rune helps to penetrate the true essence of things as well as to feel the deep intentions and motives of the people around. It is the rune of self-knowledge and introspection. It is also the rune of subtle practitioners: psychologists, doctors, fortune tellers, etc. The rune is an intermediary between consciousness and subconscious. It is usually used for successful practice with resource energy runes such as stream, power and affluence.

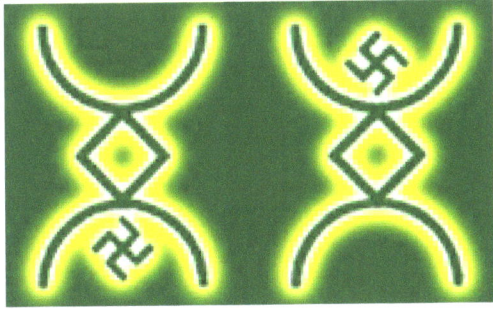

22. Runes Acceleration and Slowdown

These are the runes that set our minds to an accelerated or sloweddown mode of operation. However, when practicing with these, one should always remember that the process of acceleration or deceleration will have to be balanced by its opposite. Acceleration requires tremendous energy investment, while long deceleration can lead to stagnation. Practice with these runes is useful in the fast-track need, when a lot depends on the speed of decision-making or the speed of reaction. In other cases, the slowdown is also beneficial in force majeure situations, when events occur very quickly, and the mind is not able to cope with the psychological stress. In any case, practice with these runes requires awareness and caution so as to achieve the right outcome.

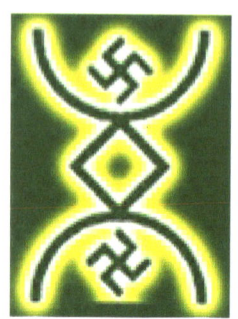

23. Rune Fire

It is the rune of the element of Fire. It is also the rune of inspiration, purification, burning and optimism. Practice with it awakens in the sub-conscious mind the desire to be visible (as opposed to the desire to hide and enclose oneself from the world). In almost every philosophical and religious doctrine, fire has been addressed as a mediator between the spiritual and earthly worlds. It is believed that in the human body, fire lives in the Manipur chakra of the solar plexus, which is responsible for social connections and success. Constant practice with this rune helps to free a person from socially restrictive programs. The practice of this rune open in a person the desire to realize the inherent talents and use them for further development.

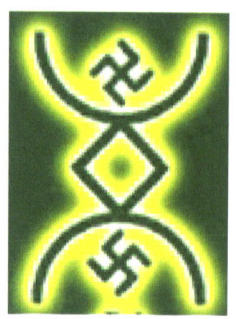

24. Rune Ice

Rune Ice is the most often used protective rune. Practice with it can be useful when the process requires stopping and rethinking about the course of action. We very often ignore and fear this state, and yet without drawing conclusions from the previous cycle, we are very likely to introduce the same mistakes and hurdles into the next. Practice with this rune often makes it possible to realize the tremendous energy resource hidden in the state of death, as a transition from one stage to another.

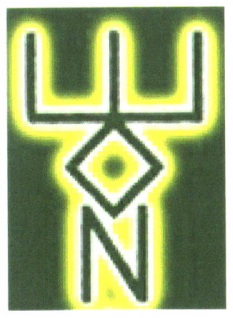

25. Rune Liberation from Lies (Disinformation)

This rune helps in getting rid of lies, manipulation and any other negative influence, especially misinformation. It is the most powerful protective and cleansing rune. Any subtle work usually begins with the practice of purification, restoration, filling, etc. Thus, it is worth starting the purification and healing of almost any life process with this rune of liberation from disinformation. It can help against stagnation, immobility in some state, fears, phobia, and it is especially useful when the state is "muddy" (the movement seems to be happening, however, it seems that there are no results, etc.). Practice of this rune is remarkably successful in situations where there is a push or imposition of someone else's opinion, however, there is no strength in the person to resist these alien influences. Also, the mental distinction between yourself and an aggressive-minded person achieved with the help of a screen from these runes helps to regain your strength and will.

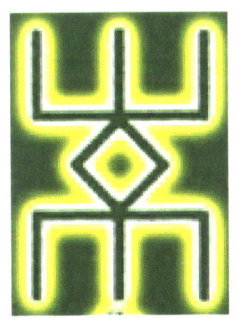

26. Rune Destruction or Purification

This rune, like rune Disinformation, carries powerful cleansing energies. However, the rune Purification on a subconscious level acts as a total disintegrator. It sets up the psyche to completely get rid of old forms and programs, no matter how useful or useless they were. This is the rune of the obsolete death. Practice with it can be very useful when there is an urgent need to start life "from a scratch", and a part of the psyche frantically grabs onto the familiar outlines, even if they have long been destructive rather than creative. This rune is also very useful to apply in cases where we feel caught in various kinds of dependencies, which usually rarely allow us to rebuild. More often, it allows natural processes to erect more productive life forms.

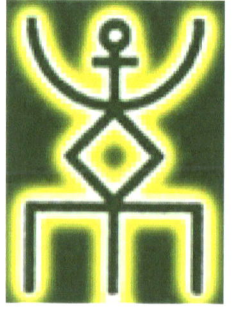

27. Rune Power or Energy

This is the rune of energy and strength. Practice with it supplies a person with an energy resource that he can direct in the desired direction. Practice with it can be invaluable when accumulation and manifestation of physical strength is required. It is the rune of sports, which helps withstand great physical exertion.

It is, thus, a rune carrying a resource for physical survival. Often in practice, this rune is used together with other runes, as an element of reinforcement, for example, runes of power, prosperity, recovery, etc.

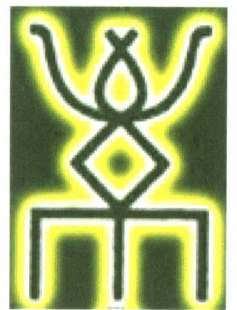

28. Rune Restorer or Recovery

This rune is the main healer of the entire rune row. Its structure consists of two parts: the upper, spiritual, symbolizing love, whereas the lower, earth, symbolizing purification. In practice, it manifests itself accordingly as painful processes requiring revision and release, followed by the filling of a new energy of creation.

It is also a rune of restoration of the primary structure. It is very often used as first aid after aggressive or negative influences.

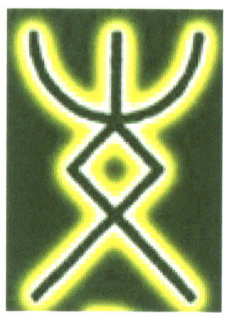

29. Rune Joy

This is the rune of joyful excitement, not only at the level of mental thought forms called positive thinking, but also at the physical bodily level. Practice with it excites a wave-like energy response in the body that stimulates movement, action and creation. This rune can be of invaluable help to lecturers, teachers and public people, whose task is to inspire others. Rune Joy stimulates in a person such energy, which is sometimes also called charisma. However, this condition, especially if it is not rooted inside (due to injuries or a weak energy system), requires a tremendous energy resource, thus, this rune is used together with rune Stream or rune Power.

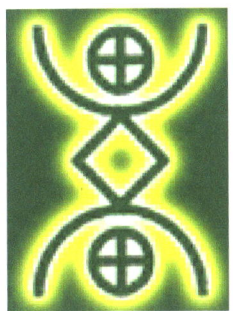

30. Rune Eternity

Rune Eternity is rarely used in everyday practice. More often, people, who have been practicing for a long time or who feel the need for knowledge of big processes, turn to it. This is the rune of meditation, inner freedom and trust. Many practices aimed at reducing the ego turn to this rune as an instrument of "dissolution in the big". Probably our consciousness does not react to any other rune with more resistance than this. It is hard for the human psyche to think that life is short and fleeting, especially against the backdrop of eras and millennia. For those who have overcome this limiting barrier of thinking, practice with rune Eternity provides a rare inspiration to rush to live and create, as long as we have the opportunity, strength and time.

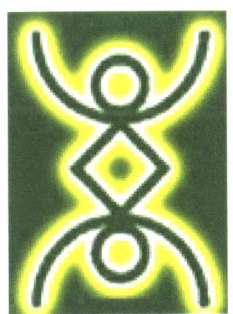

31. Rune Balance

Rune Balance, like all runes symmetrical in structure (Love, Prosperity, Awareness and Flow), helps to balance the dualities, the spiritual and material components of life. In this case, we also talk about balancing the inner and outer life of man, illusion and reality. For example, a person assimilates from childhood some kind of flawed set of ideals and requirements for himself and painfully tries to conform to them, while the reality constantly shows him that the world is ambiguous, and good often turns evil and vice versa. Practice with rune Balance helps to gradually smooth out the black and white perception and perceive the world from a position of agreement and fullness. The processes of reconciliation and balancing distortions are also remarkably straightened with the help of equilibrium energy. The voids are filled, and the excess is balanced.

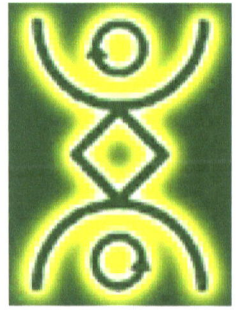

32. Rune Zero

This rune has another unspoken name - Bereginya. This is primarily a protective rune. Practice with it allows one to become uninteresting and invisible for external influences. In the normal state, we vibrate at a variety of frequencies, which is a reflection of the numerous physical and mental processes within us. These vibrations in a natural way can be caught outside where they diverge from us as a source of disturbance. The structure of the rune Zero is such that it swirls our vibrations around us so that they create an outer impermeable layer. Practice with this rune is good when we want to relax for a while and as if to fall out of the outside world. This is also the rune of peace and protected rest.

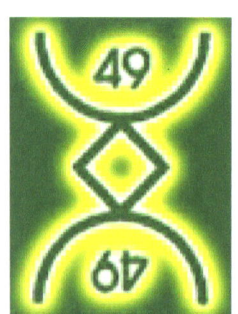

33. Rune Shell

This is the rune of our borders. Practice with it is extremely important in cases where a person feels completely unprotected and vulnerable to the outside world. Our borders are often violated or are inadequate (too weak or too impenetrable) due to childhood experiences. These can create a lot of challenges in adulthood, such as the inability to say "no" or trust someone close to you. Practice with a rune Shell allows a person to consciously adjust the permeability of the borders so that he himself feels comfortable in them.

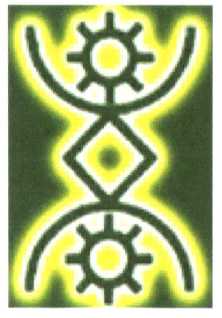

34. Rune Clarity

It is the rune of clarification and understanding. It is also the rune of openness and manifestation. Practice with it is extremely useful when the situation is ambiguous and muddy, posing difficulties to separate the main from the secondary. In the head, there is a peculiar mess of thoughts and aspirations. Rune Clarity helps to see what is happening in the sunlight, after which further actions very often become apparent. This rune is a friend of the researchers and teachers. It helps to understand the processes and patterns, along with helping to adequately and simply convey these to the listener.

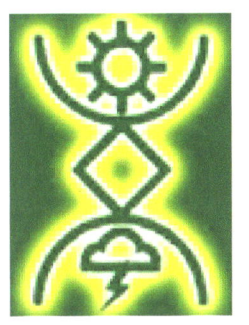

35. Rune Cloudy

This is the rune of the transitional state. Practice with it helps to undergo transitions as gently and carefully as possible for the psyche. It is used in processes when the old has become obsolete but is not completely gone, and the new is still in its infancy and takes time to fully form. Usually these conditions are very painful for our mind, as the end result is not clear and control is almost impossible. Practice with a rune Cloudy helps to find the shore or the point of support on which one can rely in a state of uncertainty and sometimes helplessness.

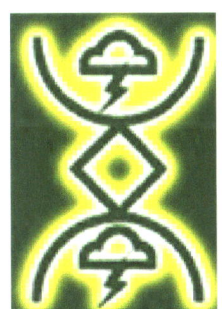

36. Rune Rain

This is the rune of purification, softening and turning inward. Practice with it can be very useful when the tension in some situations reaches the limit, and the adequacy of perception becomes dull as a result. The rune Rain creates inside a state of healthy indifference, where the tension rolls off our shoulders, like raindrops from a lotus leaf. It helps to move from a state of convulsive search for a solution to a state of conscious liberation from the need to make a decision, until the body has accumulated a sufficient resource and is ready to act. Everything has its own time - this is the blissful state that often comes with practice. Also, the rune Rain brings new life to those processes that are directed outside to the detriment of the inner life. For example, a person may be trying for years to build a life similar to "other people", without paying attention to the needs of the soul and heart, which though do not bring immediate profit, security or success, however, are needed to live. Practice with a rune of rain allows one to see these needs and provide sufficient energy for implementation. This also enables people to convert their hobbies into much more profitable businesses as compared to traditional work and career building.

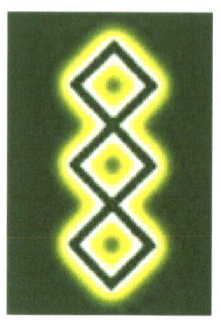

37. Rune Key

This rune symbolizes the masculine hypostasis of the rune Water. People can turn to this rune when the process is hopelessly without movement, despite the fact that there is an internal tension as well as the energy for implementation. It is, thus, not clear what steps to take and in which way to move. Practice with this rune allows one to find ways of energy output for the realization of what is planned.

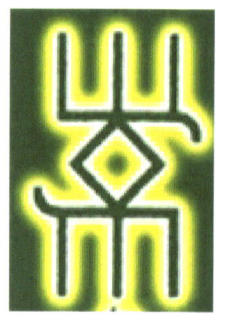

38. Rune Help

This rune is addressed when a person needs immediate assistance. Practice with it helps to find ways to come out of such situations. It also alleviates internal panic and allows one to look at things soberly. This is the rune of discovering the internal reserves of energy. From my own experience, I can say that this rune rarely "delivers", rather it provides a clear understanding of what needs to be done. Obviously, it completely depends on the person whether to do or not to do it.

5

Mandalotherapy in Practice

Do to understand ...

Any psychological therapy is not a magic pill, which we can swallow and wait for it to work. Without a doubt, miracles happen, however, as a rule, they happen exactly when a person is ALREADY trying to help himself. Thus, the person is already spending his energy, time and attention on the effort. Mandalotherapy is no exception to this rule, especially considering that the healing work is not at the level of the mind, where some complex mechanisms can be explained in simple language, but at the level of a person's energy. In most cases, it is much easier to understand than to do precisely as we are driven not by the set mental goals, but by subconscious needs. They very often differ significantly from the realized ones. For example, a person in childhood did not have enough attention from his mother, and he learned that it is possible to attract her exclusive attention by achieving some significant success. Growing up, such a person will constantly strive upwards, not for himself, but for the mother, thus, carrying a very deeply embedded destructive program. Deliberately gaining access to these programs is very difficult, as they are "sewn" into the personality from the early childhood where critical comprehension is not fully developed. Energy is both easy and difficult to work with. It is easy because one can bypass psychological defenses. It is difficult because change cannot be controlled. The movements of the soul are slow, as the wise say. Therefore, it is difficult for a Western person who is tuned in for a quick and bright result to maintain motivation in practice, especially when the results are not immediately visible. Alas, the ancient story of a lumberjack who cuts trees with a blunt ax but does not want to be distracted by sharpening his tool, is everyday's truth. Meanwhile, the results achieved while working with mandalas are not only very profound, but also have a cumulative effect. The psyche and energy change gradually, and, at some point, there is a transition from quantity to quality, making the person to suddenly realize that the problem has already been solved. My first experience with runes was exactly the same. At that stage, I still had no idea what rune influences were, and how to handle them, but being a biophysicist and an experimentalist, I decided to try "the hopeless one". At that time, I had an unfinished project on my desk, which had been in complete stagnation for two years. The initial project results were very interesting and promising, however, I didn't have the knowledge and resources to investigate the phenomenon deeply, or rather it seemed to me so. The research field was completely new, and there were only a few published works to rely on for understanding. To try my luck with runes, I laid out in a room an almost two-meter rune Growth **(Illus. 1)** carrying the energy of development (judging by the description) and stood at its center.

The sensations were very pleasant and strange. The body hummed, the fingertips vibrated, and the brain said, "it can't be". From time to time, I continued to stand at the center of the rune and "forgot" the unfinished project for a while. Two weeks later, I "accidentally" came across a project-related article which stimulated me to make a few more measurements. The results were so overwhelming that it suddenly became obvious where the attention should be directed for further research. Two months later, the project was completely accomplished, and a couple of months later, I published two articles on this topic. Only then, I realized that a miracle had happened. The cause of the problem was clearly not my inability to do something new, but the deep self-doubt. It completely changed my sense of self. I have now been practicing with runes for more than ten years. During this time, I have experienced more than sufficient evidence of the effectiveness of this practice. The life has changed completely. I have left my hired job, opened my own business, learned a new craft as a jeweler from scratch and changed my country of residence. These changes seem like as if they are driven by an invisible force. First, the internal state changed, which led to a clear understanding of the situation.

I have described the alleged mechanisms of the effect of the rune resonators on humans in previous chapters. In short, the runic structure (mandalas or single runes) evokes a resonant response inside a person, thus, rebuilding the energy in compliance with a certain reference energy source. As the resonator is not a perpetual motion machine, it transforms the energy that a person already has, thus, not only introducing a new state, but also weakening the old destructive one. There are many ways to work with rune resonators. It is important to remember that we do not influence the world and other people around us. Instead, we aim to influence our own subconscious, which is rebuilt in such a way that a solution to the problem becomes possible. Trying to influence other people with this method in order to change them for our convenience is not worth it, as there will be no effect of this method in this case. Healing and development take place only in case of personal resonance between the practitioner and practice. An important question arises at the point, "where to begin?"

The practice of laying out runes and mandalas

This is one of the best ways to feel the subtle energy of runes and mandalas physically, so to speak, at the level of sensations in the body. It helps to distinguish between the features of impact and range of applicability of a particular rune. Usually, after the first practice, a person can track the result of exposure and decide whether he should move in this direction or look for something else. Spreading runes and mandalas in nature **(Illus. 2)** is an effective alternative, ideally in places of power (places located in geoactive zones where we can feel a surge of strength). Both mandalas and runes are best laid out with natural materials. These can be spread with stones, grain or cereals, cones, chestnuts or twigs. One can use fruits, vegetables or nuts (a wonderful practice during the

season of ripening of the gifts of nature in one's own garden, if any).
After this practice, the vegetables and fruits can and should be eat-
en, as they are very beneficial for the body. It is worth starting to lay
out individual runes first, followed by mandalas. Runes should be
laid out starting from the central square, followed by laying out the
outline clockwise, starting from the left horizontal vertex. Usually,
the ideal rune size is from a meter or more, so that one has the opportunity to stand in the center of the laid-out rune, or even better
to sit in meditation. It is the best if one can lie down and relax in the
center. One can choose any rune to lay out. If there are no priorities,
it is better to start with the rune Purification and Destruction **(Illus.
3)**.

After the rune is laid out, one should stand in the middle of the central square and take several deep breaths and exhalations to relax.
The more relaxed our body is, and the more we are in contact with
it, the easier it is to feel the energetic influence of the rune oscillatory circuit. In cases where it is difficult to relax, and one practically
does not feel anything, the rune can be made under the bed. Alter-
natively, a large rune can be made from cardboard, by securing
grain or pebbles with glue. The more voluminous is the contour, the
stronger is the response, in general. Such a rune can be pushed under the bed at night, whereas it can be taken out during the day to
work with it if there is time. The advantages of the rune over which
one can lie include the maximum relaxation and ability to listen
freely to the sensations in the body. Once one gets comfortable with
laying out runes, it can be followed by with laying of mandalas. As
compared to runes, the energy of the mandalas is more powerful,
and changes in the subconscious are faster. One should always remember that when energy begins to circulate through the body, the
first thing that happens is the cleansing of the channels. This can be
expressed in pop-up memories, feelings of slight discomfort in
those areas where energy cannot pass freely, rising fears, etc. However, all of these discomforts are short-term. It is important not to
keep everything floating up or suppress it again, but to allow it to

freely leave the body, thus, to become absolutely conducted for this energy and agree with everything that rises. Regular practice helps to remove the initial barriers in the flow of energy, and the body learns to immediately absorb the resource energy and recharge.

Practice of working with runic streams to heal the body

This method is based on an ancient technique, dealing with the movement of the point of attention along the main energy channels of the body (or working with problem areas). As it is known, where there is attention, both energy and disease are there. By clearing the energy channels, we restore the primary flow of energy, and many diseases pass naturally and imperceptibly. The use of runes and runic mandalas allows one to modulate the energy of the impact, or in other words, provides the qualities necessary for each specific task. For example, at the beginning of the practice, one can use the energy of Purification and Disinformation to remove the extraneous energetic influences and cleanse the channels from "fine" dirt. Following this, one can use the energy of the rune Restoration to restore the original structure. Subsequently, the energies of filling, such as Love, Growth and Prosperity can be activated. Our task is to clearly imagine the desired rune (or mandala), mentally place it in the body and allow it to move along the paths indicated below, thus, directing it and constantly keeping our attention on it. It is possible to form a rune stream of a certain quality imagining, for example, that the required rune forms an infinite number of its small replicas, organized into one luminous stream moving along the energy meridians. The main trajectories of movement include:

Spine

It comprises of up and down as well as spiral movements along the spinal column. If, in the process of movement, any images of congestion, stuck energetic "mud" or dark inclusions (which often happens, especially when working with the energies of Purification) appear in your imagination, you should pay more attention to this place and work with it until mental energy will flow freely. Usually, if the practice is done correctly, the internal massage is accompanied by a "bath", as the body becomes hot from the released energy.

Spine - External energy boundaries

It is the movement involving both the body and personal space around it (called the Aura, the vernal borders inhabited by the bubble, or Zhilo (among the Slavs)) **(Illus. 4)**. This space unites all energy bodies of a person, including soul and spirit. The contour is a "coil" in which the energy moves up and down the spine, goes about 20-40 cm beyond the legs and head. Subsequently, it spirals in the opposite direction (up and down), moving along the outer boundaries of our energetic cocoon. This is a powerful practice of accumulating energy and deep cleansing of the energy structure of the body, if runes and cleansing mandalas are used. The main task is the same as working with spine: to clear the inner and outer space from fine dirt and restore the natural circulation of energy.

Work with the area of the unhealthy organ

The principle is the same: up-down, left-right and spiral movements, covering the entire area of an unhealthy organ. Any disease, as you know, has a physical and a psychological component. The latter component is sometimes called psychosomatics or active field dynamics, signaling a kind of psychological block that leads to the curvature of the original energy flow. Very often, when working with runes, the true reason pops up in the mind in the form of a state or emotion that needs to be seen, recognized and released.

Practice of energy work with the purpose

When the initial acquaintance with the runes has taken place, and you already "understand-feel" their energies, you can proceed to the next stage: drawing up individual rune compositions that will help in the implementation of the desired goal. For this, rune structures in the form of mandalas are ideal. Mandalas can be laid out **(Illus. 5)** or drawn. One can also use the images of mandalas, however, this approach requires some skill for concentration. In the center of the mandala, usually those runes are placed the energies of which are the most consistent with the goal. For example, if the goal is to achieve prosperity, the central runes can be Universal Wealth, Growth and Wealth, Path and Wealth, Equilibrium and Wealth, etc. In drawing up rune combinations, it is important to feel how well the runes combine with each other and if there is any contradiction in their energies. For example, cleansing runes (Cleansing, Getting rid of Lies and Scattering) rarely go well with the runes of states (Love, Equilibrium and Knowledge). Similarly, the rune Stream does not get along too well with rune Castle. There are times when such a combination is necessary due to the specificity of the request, however, in general, the stretched combinations are best avoided.

Such a runic combination is placed at the center of one of the sacred geometric structures described in the previous chapters. Such structures not only enhance the action of the central runes, but also create a certain way or path for the distribution of energy in the mandala. For example, mer-ka-ba finetunes the runic mandala to combine dualities and promotes the development of flexibility and unconditionality of the mind.

Next, the runes of the so-called second circle are selected. These are the auxiliary energies that help in the implementation of the plan. For example, if the goal is the development of a profitable business, the runes of the periphery can be Victory, Flow, Knowledge, Joy, Power, etc. Finally, the last step is to lay the outer rim of the mandala. It is responsible for the outer boundaries acting as a protective layer. Runes such as Protection, Joy, Flow, Path, Goal Setting, etc., fall adequately into the outer rim. From my own experience, the structure of a mandala should not be created with the mind, but with the heart and intuition. If, for example, there is a desire to insert one or another rune or geometric structure in the mandala, it is worth doing exactly the way you want, and not the way it is logical. The reason for the discrepancy most often lies precisely in the fact that the subconscious and conscious may have a different understanding of what we really need. From experience, a person very rarely chooses a mandala that is tuned directly to the request voiced by him. For example, he comes for the mandala of Prosperity and chooses either Growth, Protection or Love. This happens not because he does not need money, but because they mean security and opportunity to develop or attract love (here you should immediately think about the early psychological trauma of abandonment or lack of attention) for the person. In the latter case, not even the mandala of Love is optimal, rather the use of Healer or Purification is more beneficial to remove the traumatic material. Obviously, it is much easier to solve the problem if you act directly, without an "intermediary". However, our subconscious is much wiser than consciousness in many cases. Thus, if one wants love, healing of early traumas is necessary, followed by practice with growth and balance.

Practice with the Mandalas I have already made

The mandala laid out for your personal request is a very powerful tool for customization and "self-assembly". After the mandala falls into your hands, it must be cleaned of all extraneous energies, except directly the energy of the runic structures **(Illus. 6)**. You can put a candle in the center of the mandala or can light incense sticks and fumigate the mandala with their fragrant smoke. You can put the mandala in the sun for a while. Subsequently, one should "put" one's intention into the center of the mandala and assign a task to the instrument. Although, it would be more correct, of course, to say - to set a task for your psyche when working with a mandala. Afterwards, it can be hung on the wall, preferably opposite or behind the place where you spend a lot of time. For example, in front of the desktop. If the mandala is large (about a meter), it is great to put it behind your back while working. In this case, the mandala works even without your active participation **(Illus. 7)**.

You can also put small mandalas under the pillow or set them at the bedhead so that the center is directed to the crown. This method works well when we need to find a solution to a difficult problem. This way, the answer may be revealed in a dream. Very often, medical professionals place the mandalas behind the client during work sessions or under the massage table. In such cases, the mandala needs to be cleaned often, of course. I want to remind once again that our intuition will tell us more clearly how to use the mandala for the maximum benefit. Every moment of life is unique and requires its own approach. Written laws are rarely effective when it comes to the human psyche. We are all different, and our states change differently depending on time and environmental conditions. The one who knows how to meet the needs of the moment wins. Try it, listen to yourself, choose what is right for you, and the results will not take long.

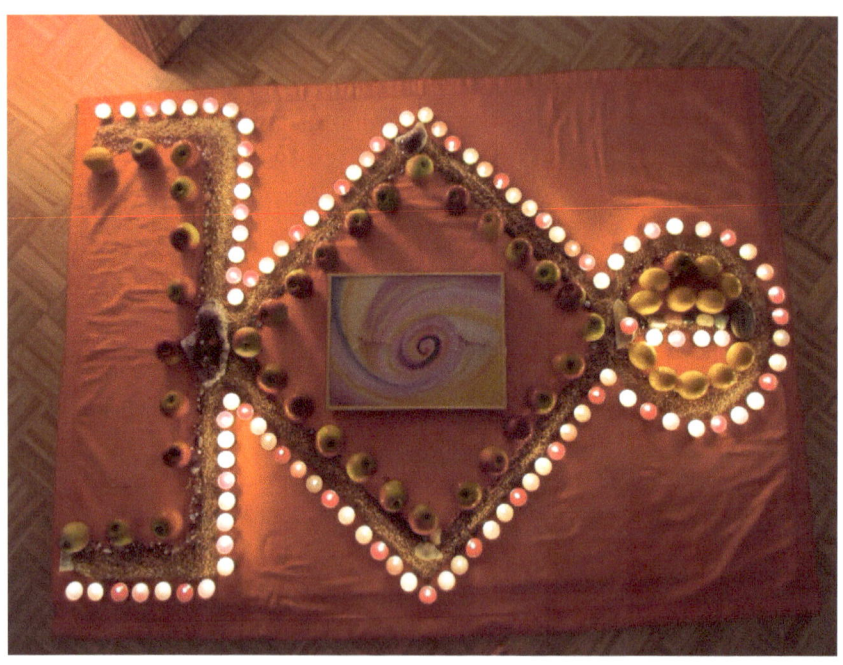

Illustration 1. *Rune Growth.*

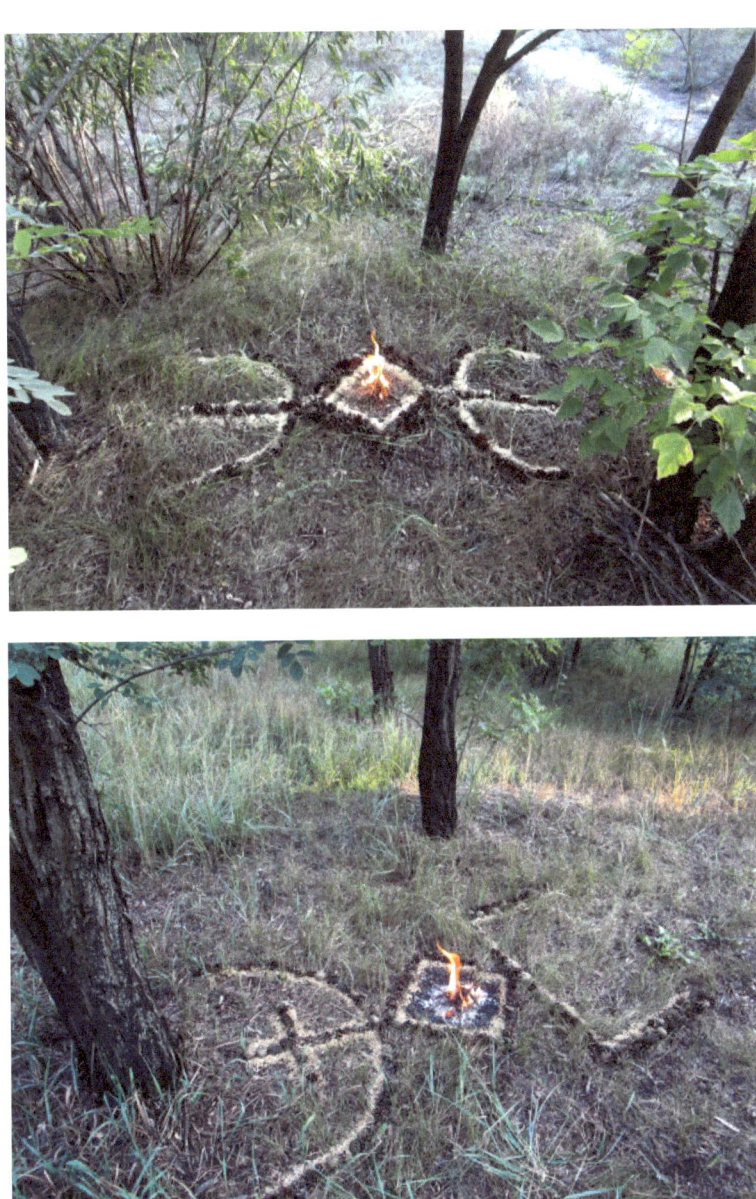

Illustration 2. *Runes Wealth and Victory, made in Nature.*

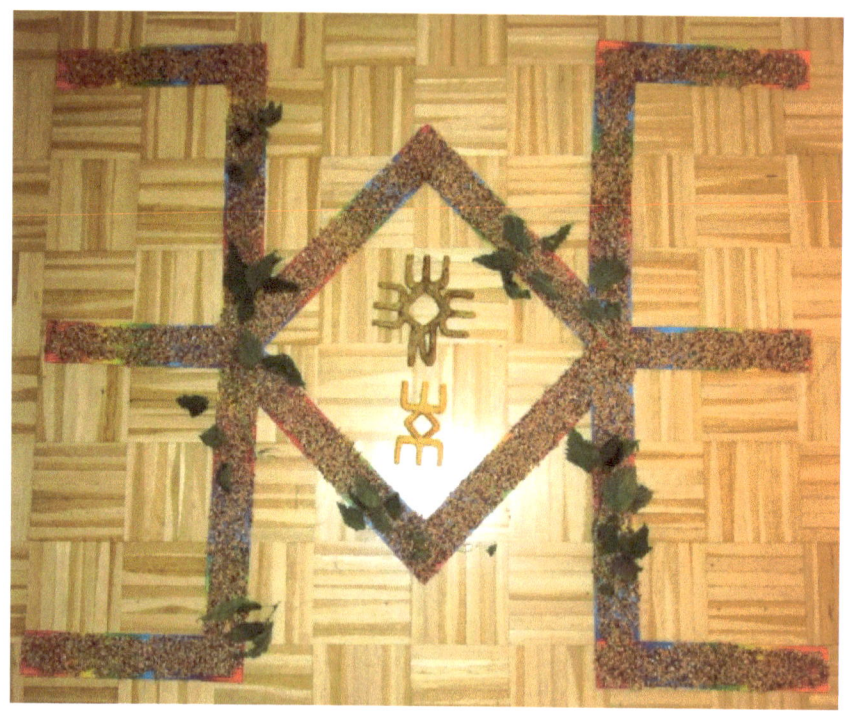

Illustration 3. *Rune Purification.*

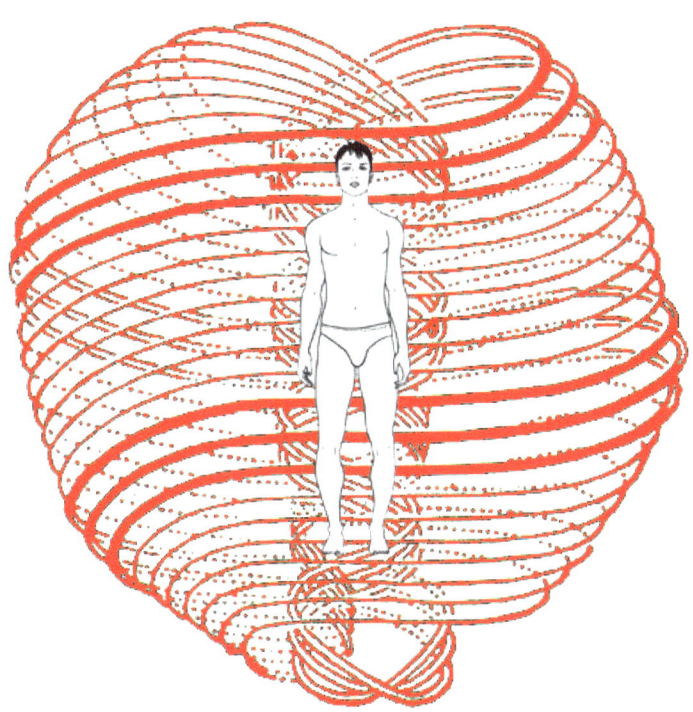

Illustration 4. *Energy lines around healthy human body.*

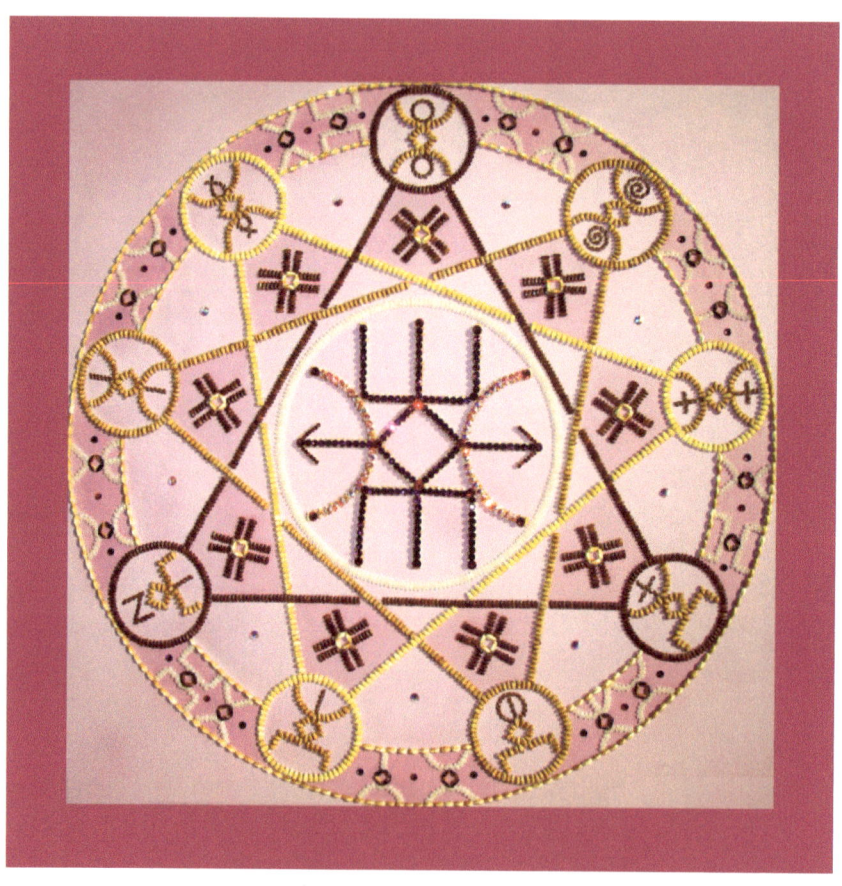

Illustration 5. *Mandala Purification and Scattering.*

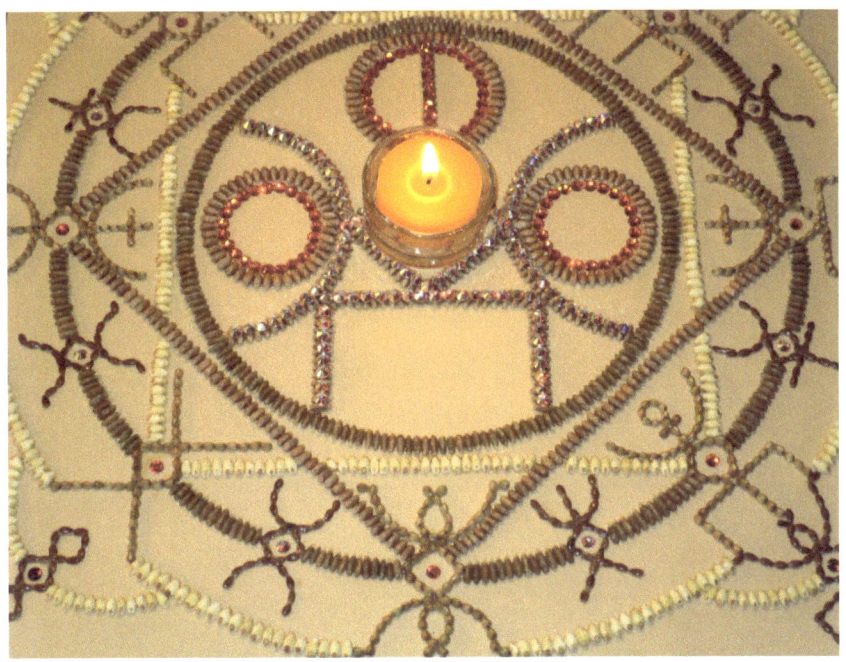

Illustration 6. *Cleaning of the mandala before practice.*

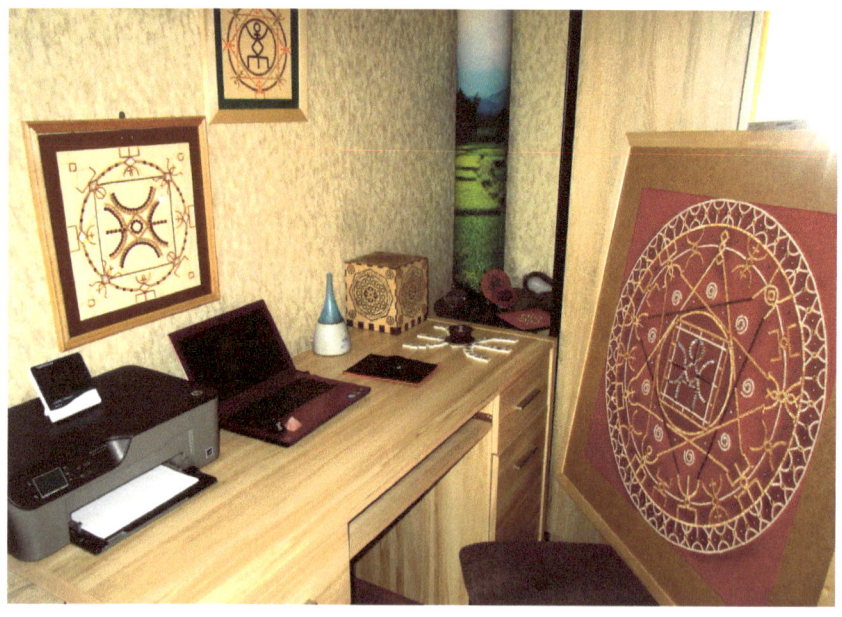

Illustration 7. *Mandalas in the working space at home.*

6

Rune Mandalas in the Form of Jewelry

Wearing body jewelry, symbolizing various forces and energies, is customary in the culture of almost every country as well as religious, social and spiritual traditions. The decoration is a kind of key to enter certain energy channels. Such channels can carry the collective energy and can also directly access natural energy sources. For example, a pectoral cross for Christians is a symbol of devotion to the Christian religious tradition. Through it, a person can enter into resonance with the energies of the so-called Christian egregor. Among the pre-Christian Slavs, the solar symbols (e.g. the solar circle), symbolizing various aspects of solar energy such as healing, protection, wisdom and fertility, were used as body jewelry. Wearing jewelry is primarily a resourceful practice. Through resonance with great forces, a person has the opportunity to connect and draw energy from the source to which the symbol is dedicated. For an individual, such a source is inexhaustible, for it is created by forces much greater than one person. Also, if a piece of jewelry has a sacred structure and is a resonator, it can transform a person's energy from one quality to another. Adept practitioners call this "configuring personal energy on the mandala". If some external conditions knock a person out of balance and lead to an internal contradiction, wearing jewelry can help "reconcile" the conflicting principles and lead to integrity. On these basic principles, i.e. access to the resource and the transforming effect, the so-called protective properties of jewelry are based. We are not protected by magical otherworldly forces, but by our own abilities, peacefully dormant until the need for them arises. The possibilities of the human psyche are orders of magnitude wider than those put in use every day. This has been vividly demonstrated more than once by practitioners and followers of various schools as well as the ordinary people who find themselves in life-threatening conditions. The problem of access to these resources in most cases is very simple - we do not need "super" abilities in everyday life, as we can perfectly manage without them. In very simple words, "power is given for the cause". The more global are the tasks befalling a person, the more energy and abilities he has. Such energy and qualities are rarely present "ready-made" from birth. More often, such abilities are acquired in the process of solving problems that go beyond the usual "consumption" of life. That is why the choice of protective jewelry is a very individual process. The disclosure of an internal resource invariably entails changes in real life. Energy requires an outlet, otherwise a person may feel uncomfortable from an excess of energy. The same is also true for the lack of energy.

The jewelry presented in this chapter has been created for different people, according to their needs and tasks. If any of the jewelry catches attention and stands out, it is worth considering. Perhaps your inner nature requires you to pay attention to these aspects of your life and to develop them. "What you are looking for is also looking for you", as Jellaladin Rumi said.

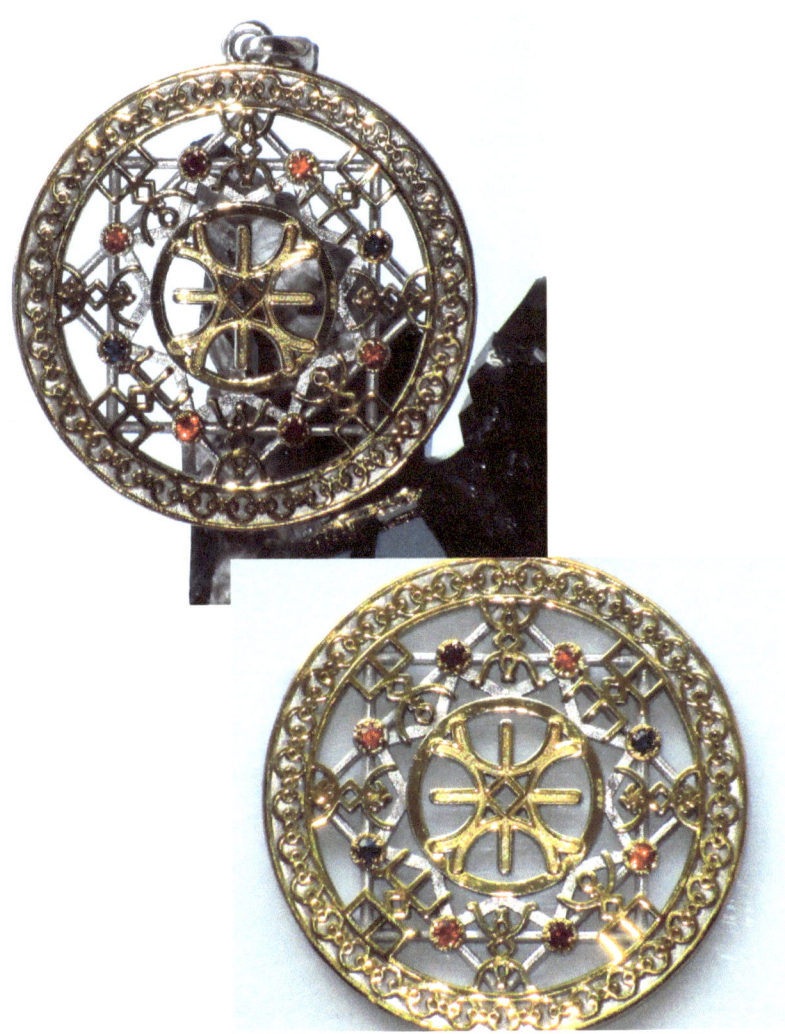

Illustration 1. *Mandala "Universal Prosperity", Created to unlock an inner state of abundance in the broadest sense of the word. An abundance of material resources, money, energy, satisfying relationships, etc.*

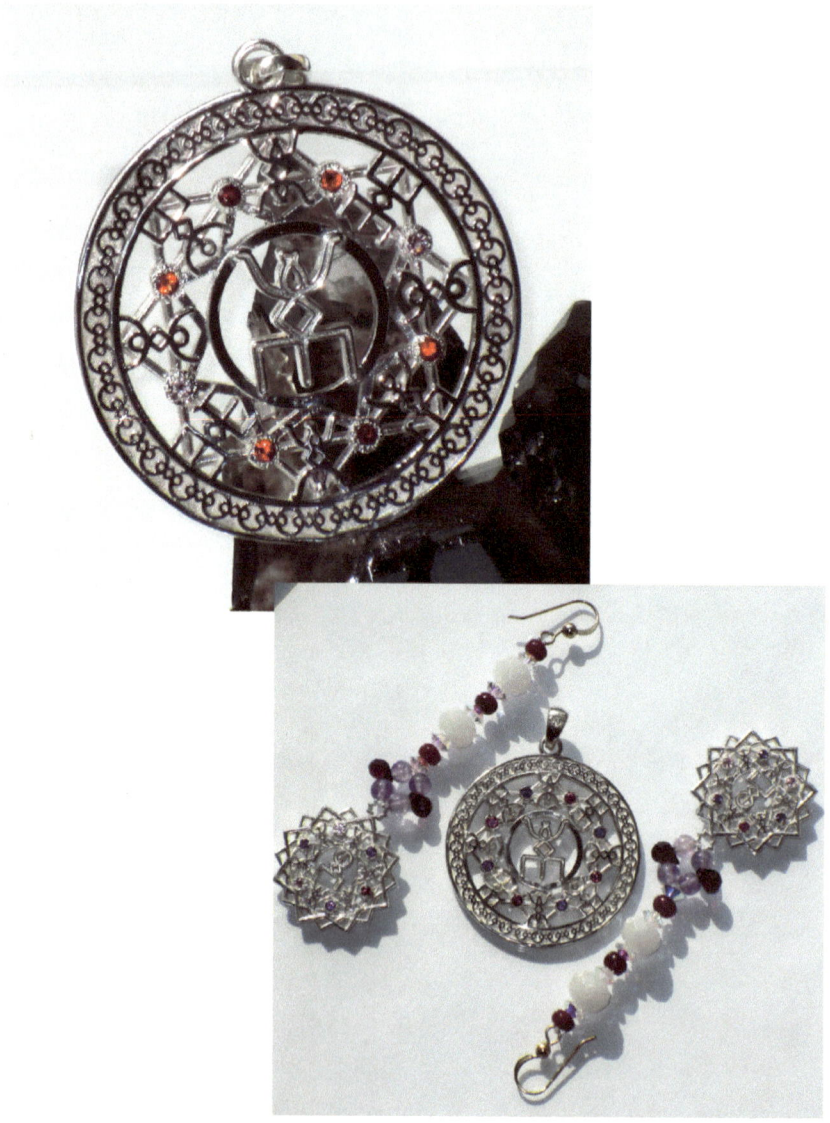

Illustration 2. *Mandala "Healer". It was created to heal the body and soul from the consequences of psychological traumas that interfere with the perception of life in its entirety. It is made of silver, rubies and sapphires.*

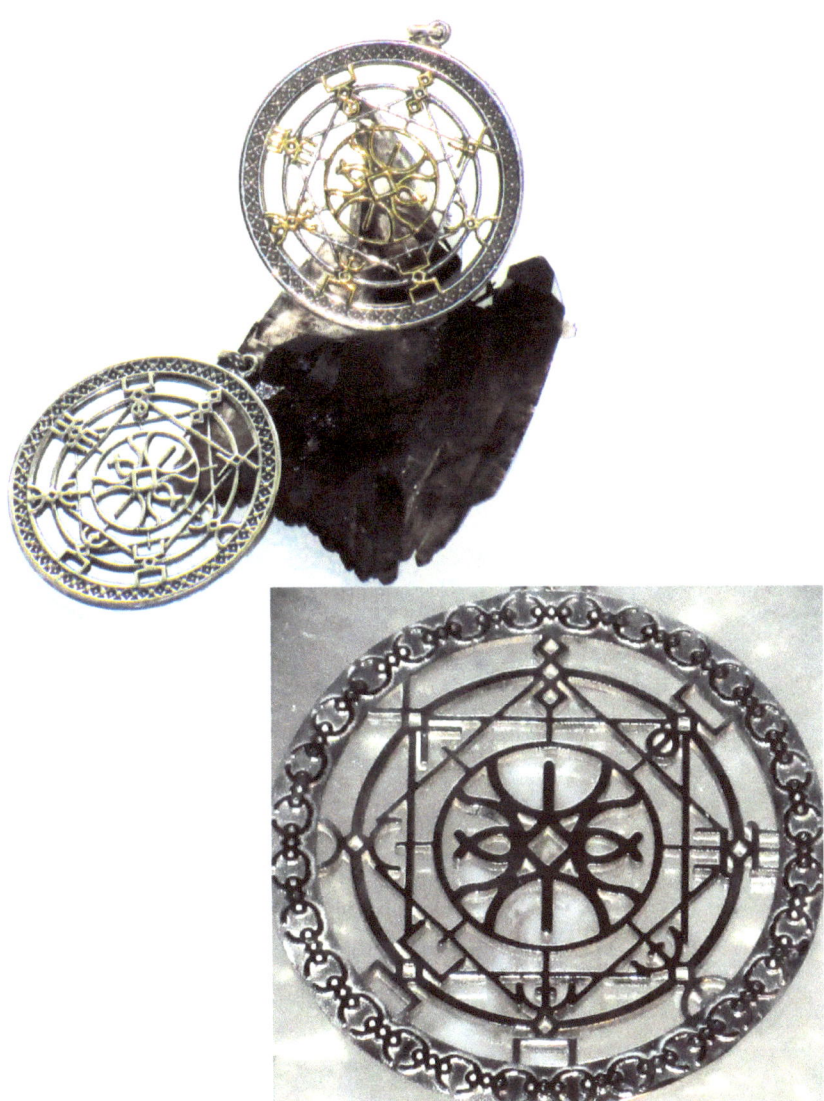

Illustration 3. *Mandala "Love and Prosperity" was created as an activator of those sides of the psyche that create harmonious relationships filled with love and mutual understanding, along with a state of inner wealth. It is made of silver with partial gilding.*

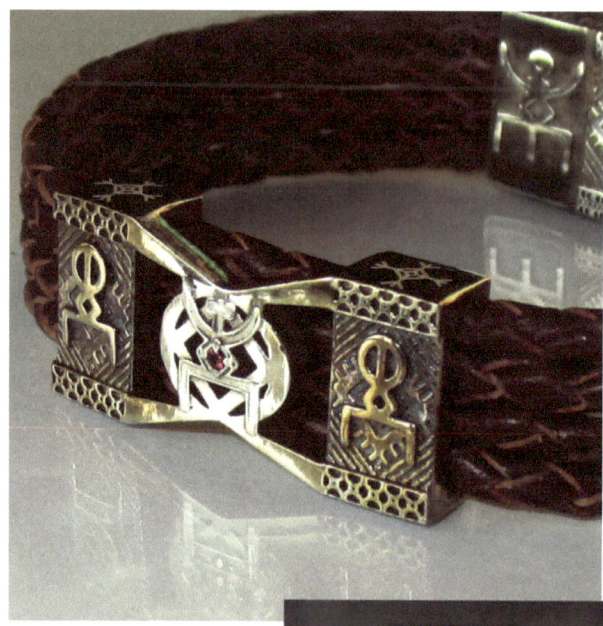

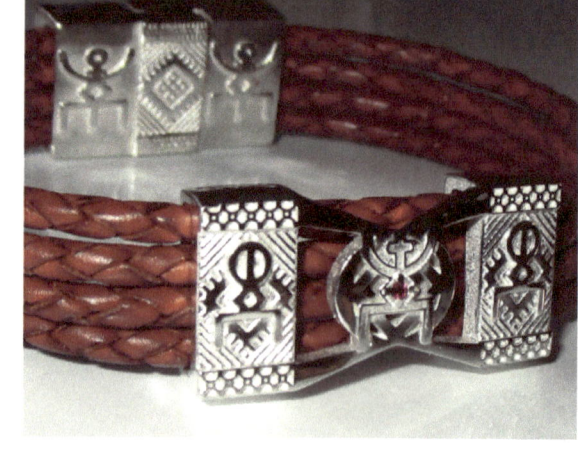

Illustration 4. *Bracelet "Development and Success". This piece of jewelry was created for a man seeking to move his business to a higher level of development, new opportunities and profitability. It is made of silver (partial artistic blackening), rubies and leather.*

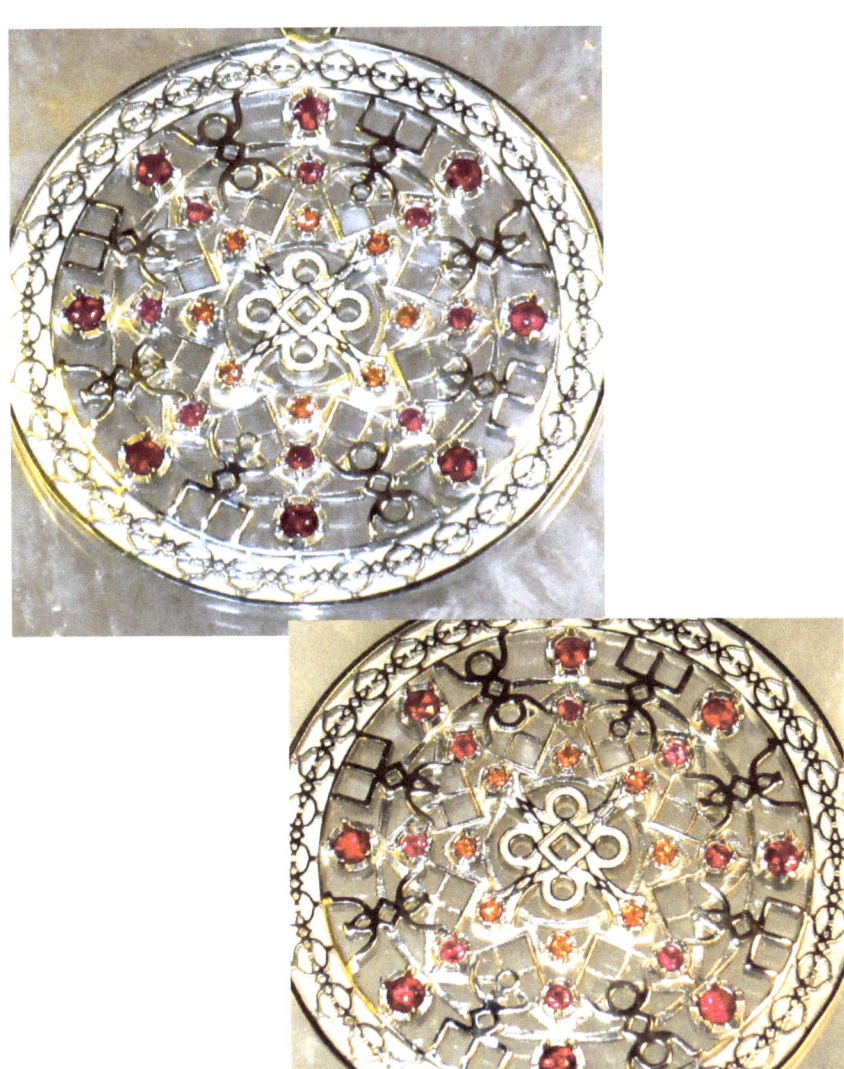

Illustration 5. *Mandala "Equilibrium" was created to help reconcile internal contradictions as well as find internal balance and harmony between material and spiritual, female and male, work and leisure, etc. It is made of silver, sapphires and rubies.*

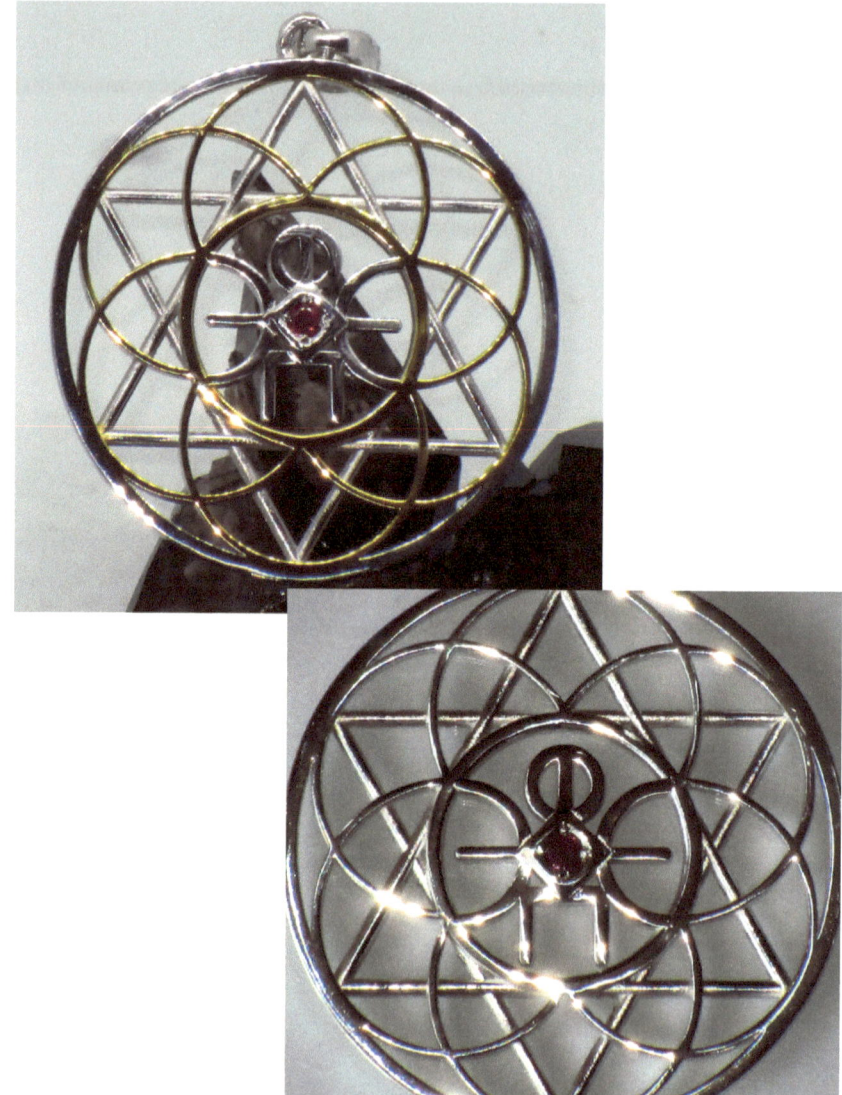

Illustration 6. *Mandala "Growth and Wealth". This jewelry was created in order to unlock a person's ability to earn money, in harmony with healthy self-expression and self-realization. It is made of silver, gilding and ruby.*

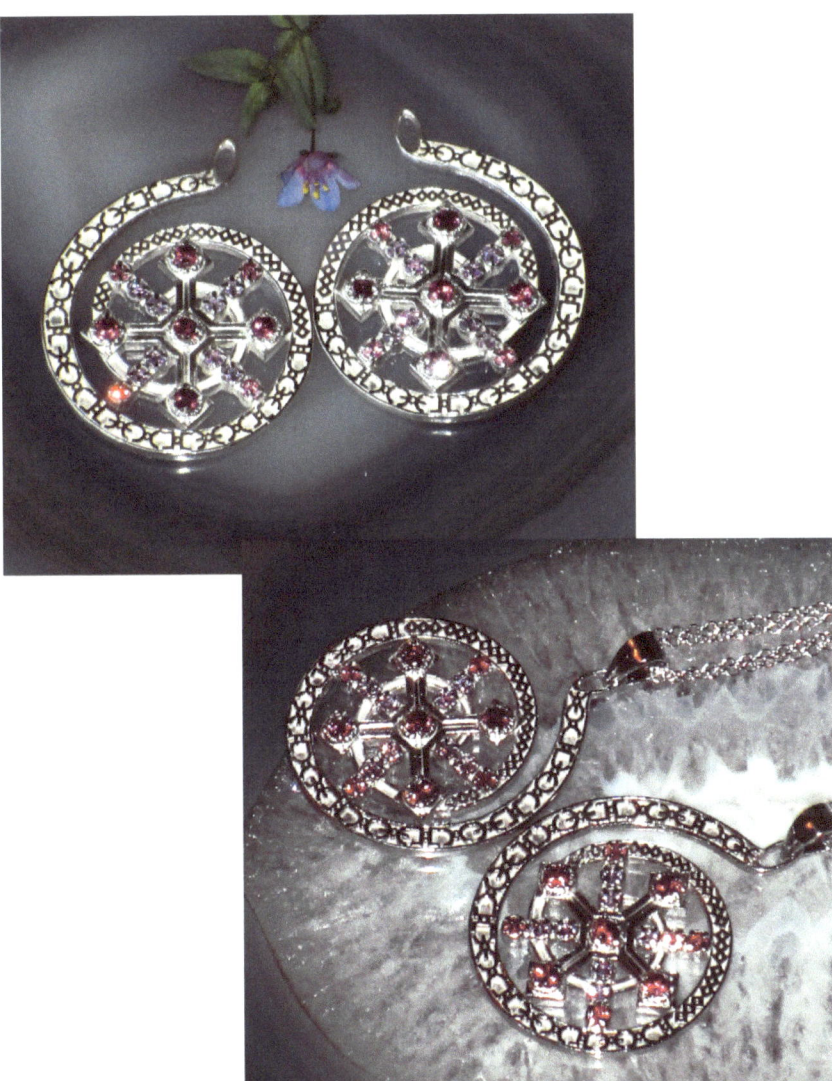

Illustration 7. *Earrings and pendant "Talent". These decorations were created in order to awaken, bring to the surface and realize the inner talents of a person. There are made of silver, sapphires, rubies, rhodolites and amethysts.*

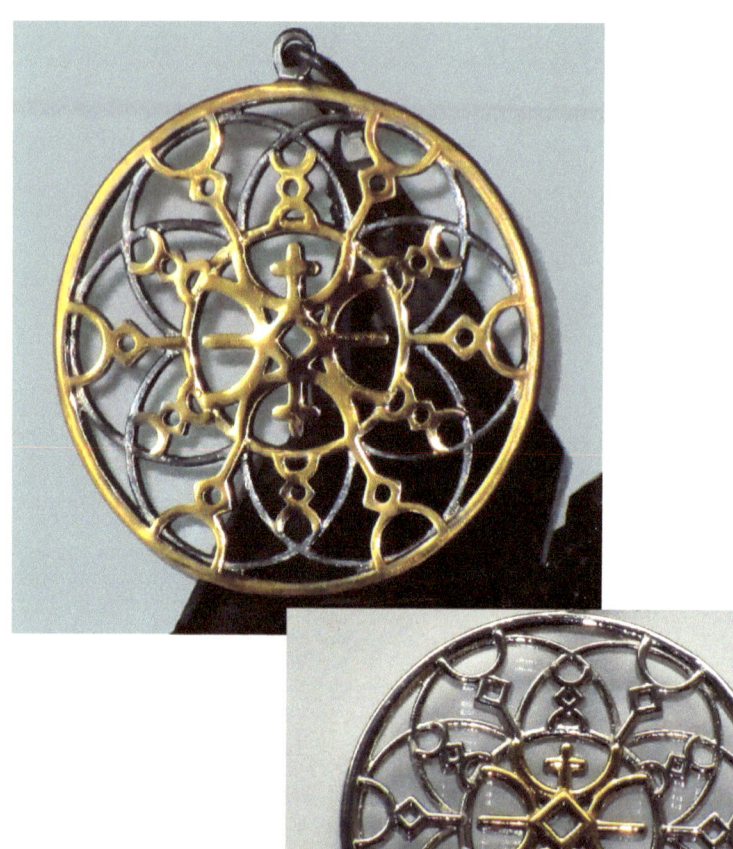

Illustration 8. *Mandala "Knowledge and Wealth". This mandala was created to enable a person to fully reveal his intuition, thus, directing him to achieve internal and external well-being. It contains silver, rhodium plating and gilding.*

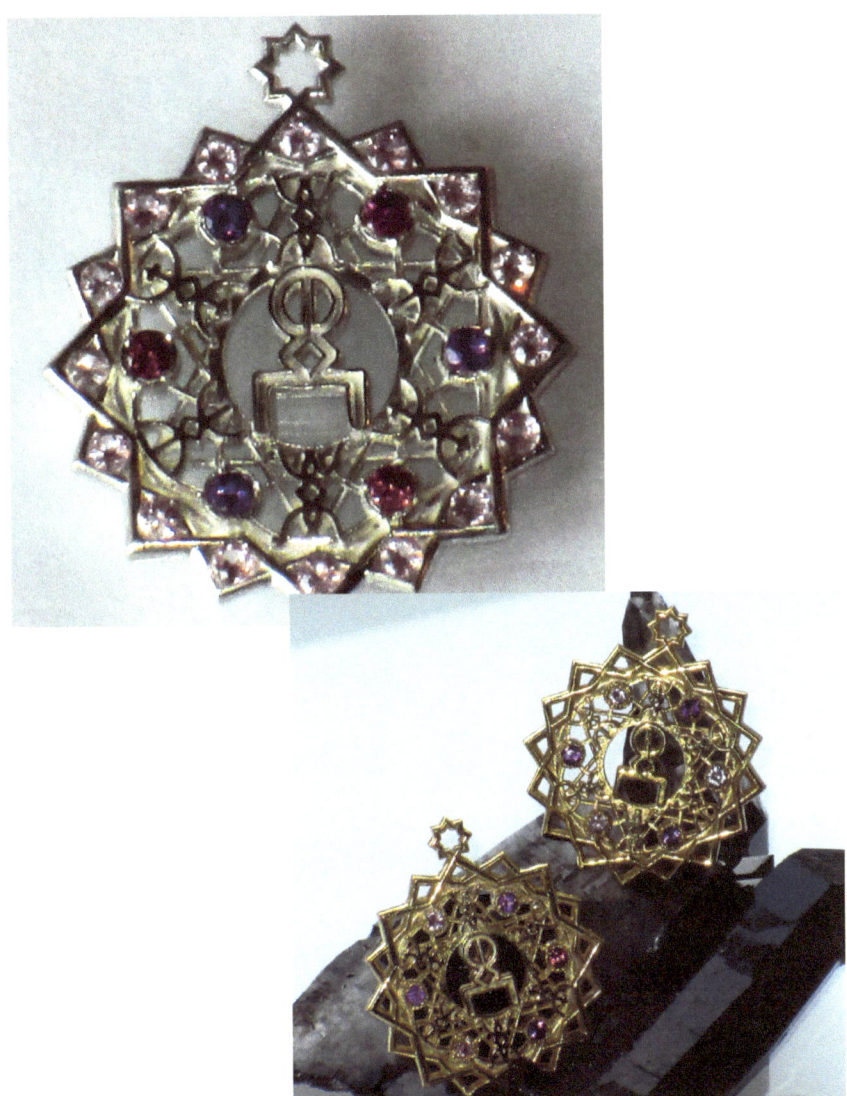

Illustration 9. *Mandala "Growth and Development". These pendants were created for people who feel stagnation in life and want to take it to a qualitatively new level. These pendants help to achieve the feeling of joy, satisfaction and harmony. These are made of silver, gold, sapphires, rhodolites and amethysts.*

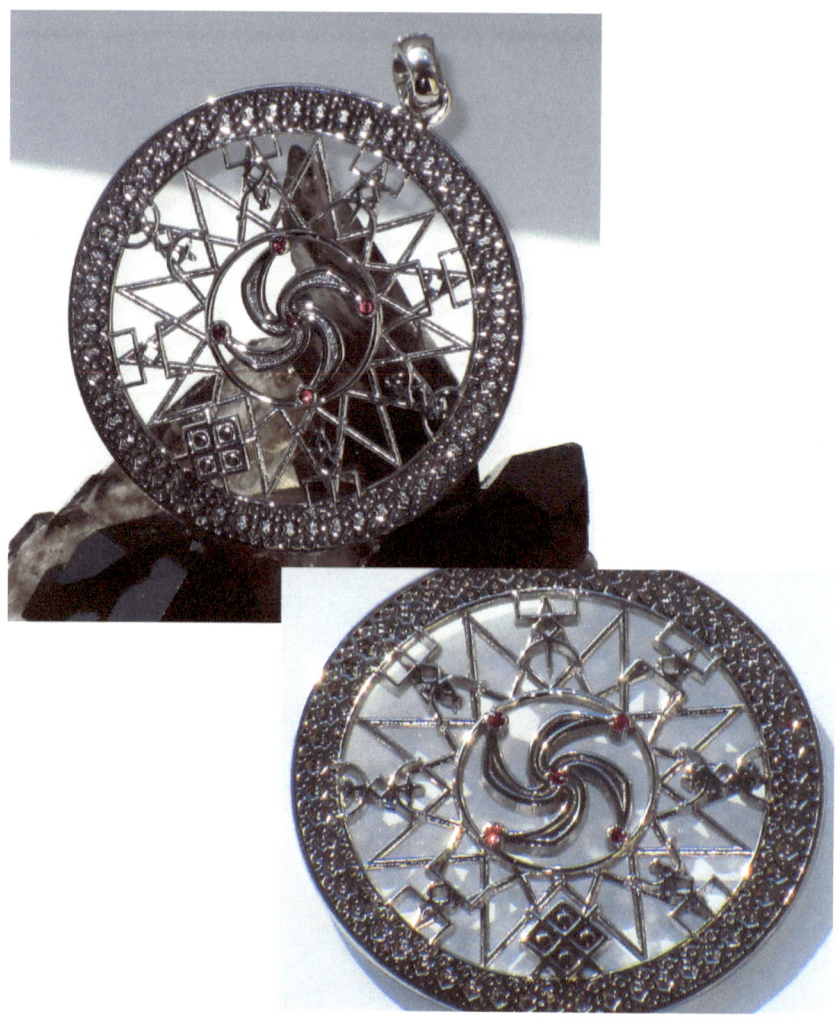

Illustration 10. *Mandala "Symbol of the Family". This mandala was created for a powerful practitioner who wants to work with resources such as the elements of nature and generic energies. It is made of silver and rubies.*

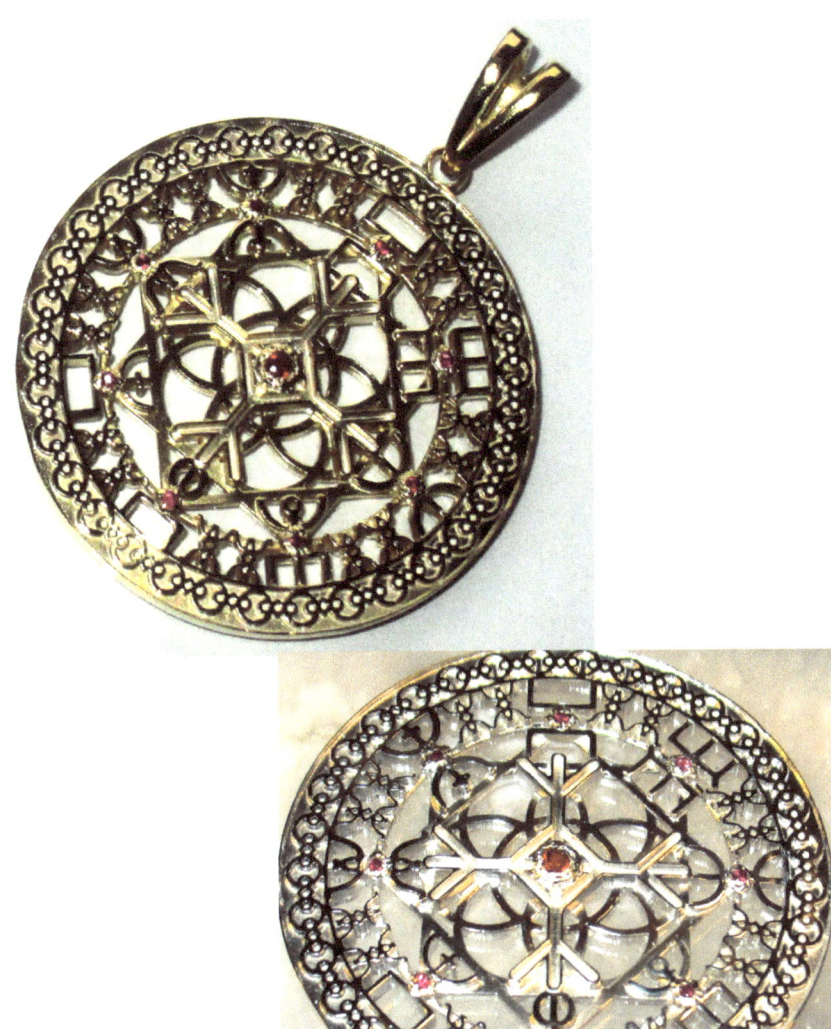

Illustration 11. Mandala "Glory" was created for a person who sets big and humane goals not only in business, but also in life. It is made of silver, gilding, rubies and sapphire.

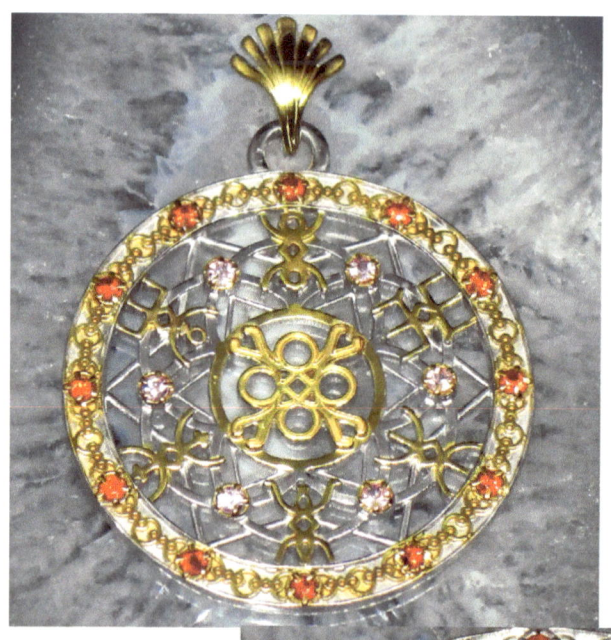

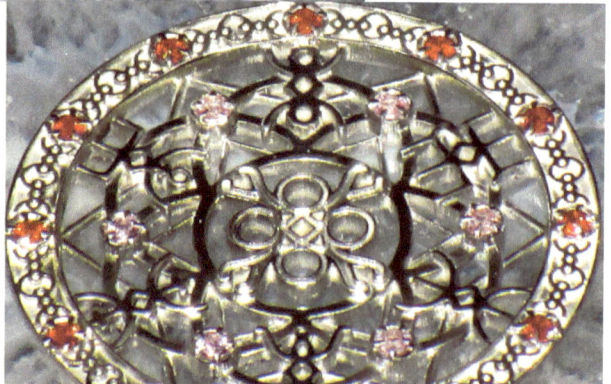

Illustration 12. *Mandala "The Force Awakens". This decoration carries in itself the spring energies of the awakening of Nature, the discovery of the feminine power and its appeal for the benefit of oneself and people. It contains silver, gilding and sapphires.*

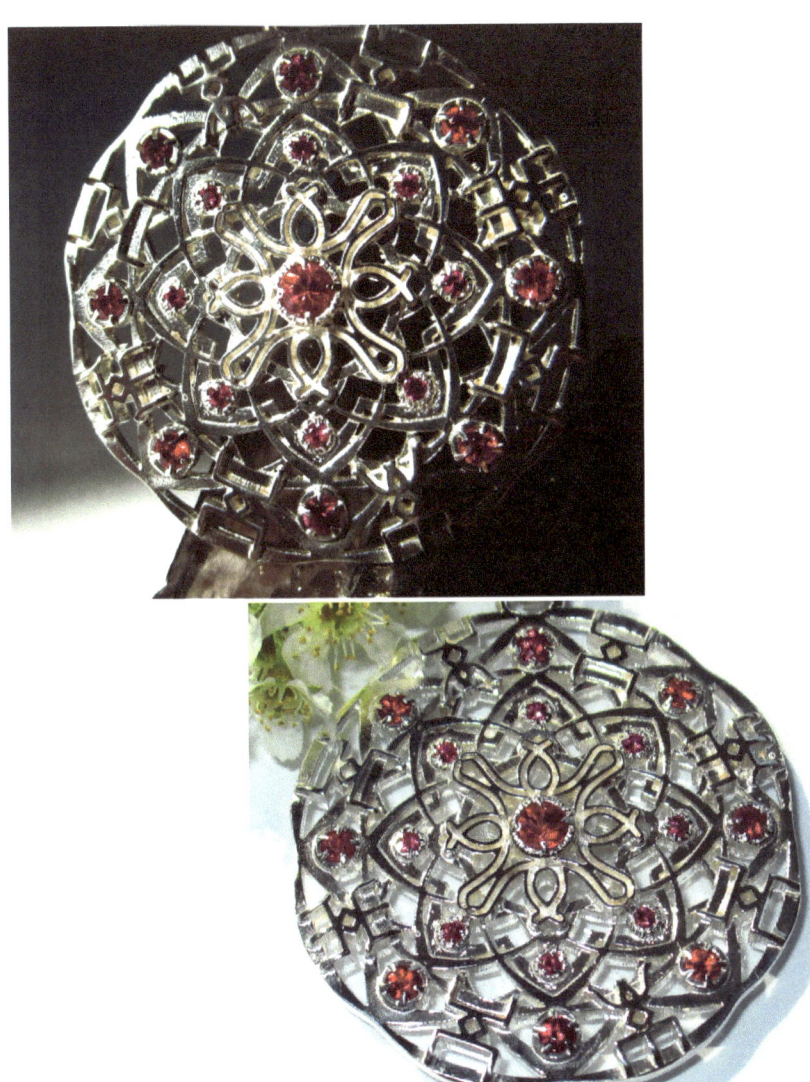

Illustration 13. *Mandala "Universal Love". It is the mandala of disclosure and connection with the universal flow of love - as a universal force for the development and creation of all living things. It is made of silver, rubies and sapphires.*

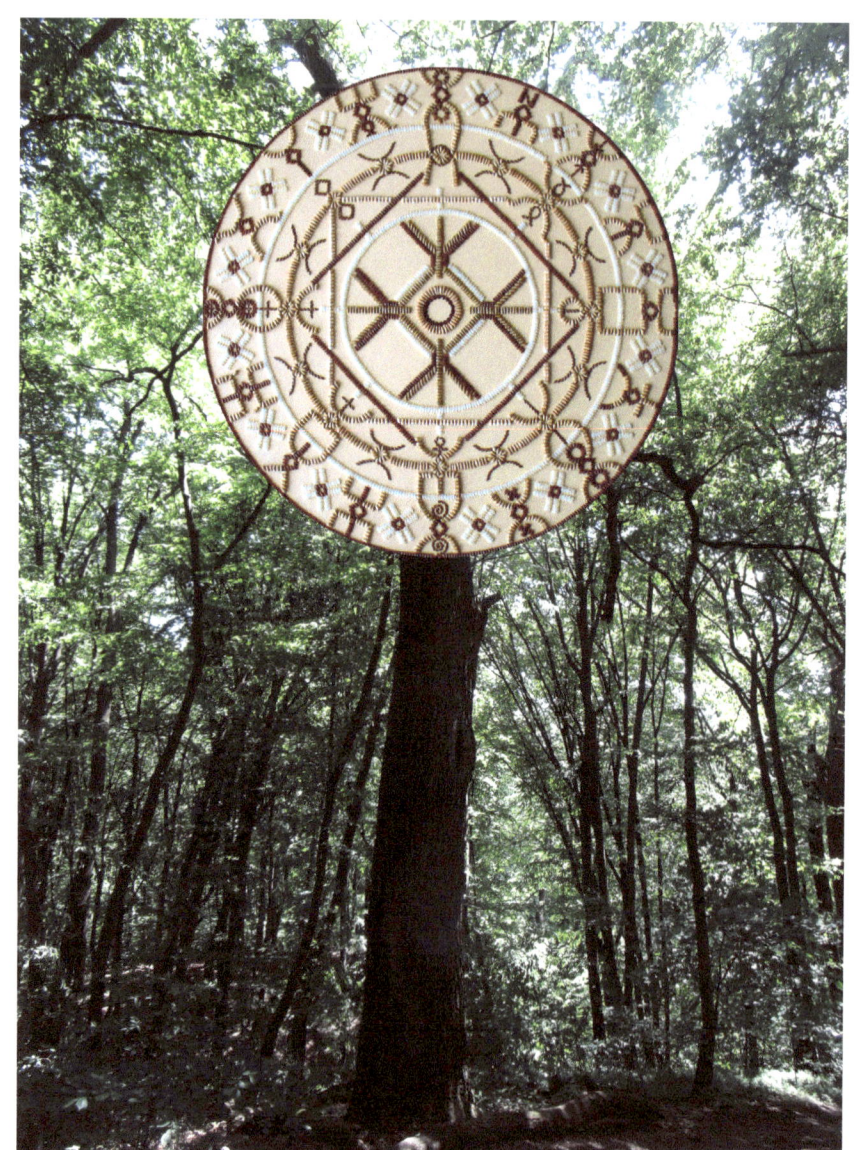

7

Rune Mandalas for Life

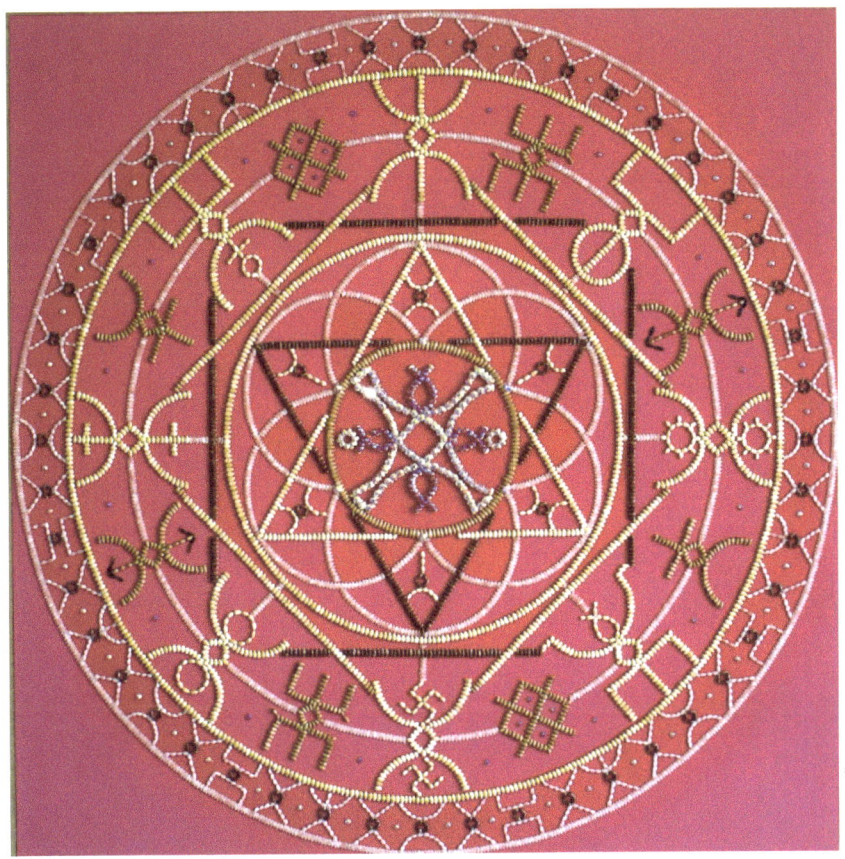

Illustration 1. *Women Hypostasis of the Universe*
The mandala of primal feminine energy. It has many names: limitless alive,
loving Earth Mother, Mary, Mom, etc. It represents not only the love and
unconditional support, but also the primal energy, power and depth. All
material goods come through it, too. It is our connection to Mother and our
energy channel with female generic resource.

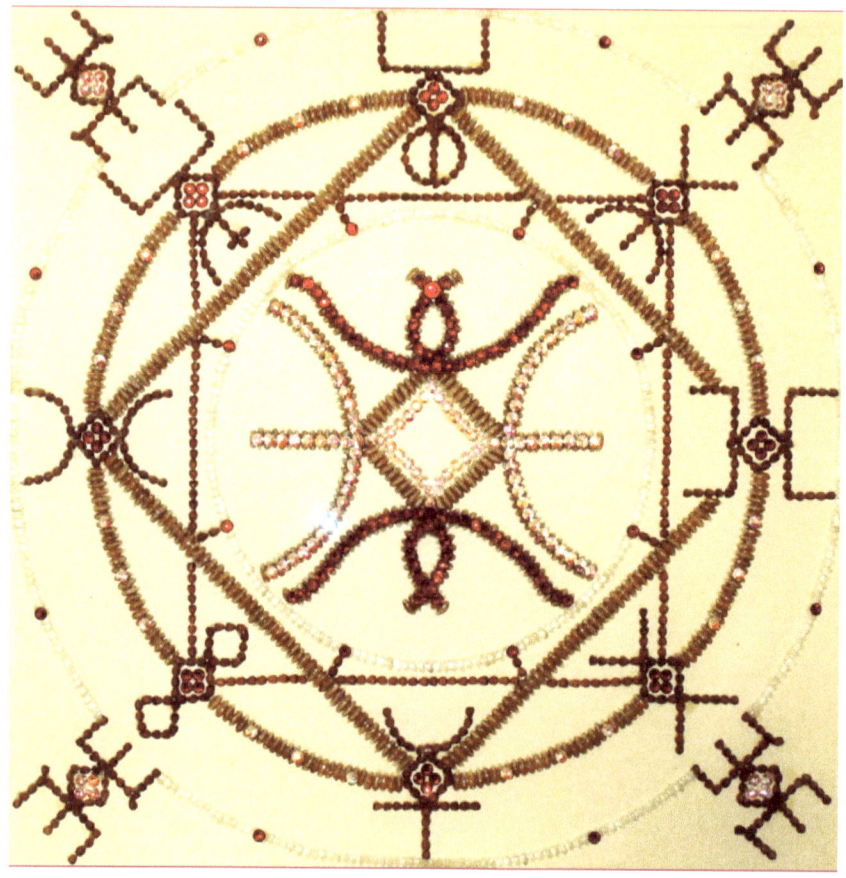

Illustration 2. *Universal Prosperity*
This mandala is a powerful activator of those sides of the soul and mind that allow a person to be in abundance (material and spiritual energies). It is no secret that the universe is by its nature abundant, and the only hurdle that prevents all these benefits from being found is in the person himself. This mandala will help not only to get rid of non-constructive attitudes, but also to attract additional external opportunities and resources into your life.

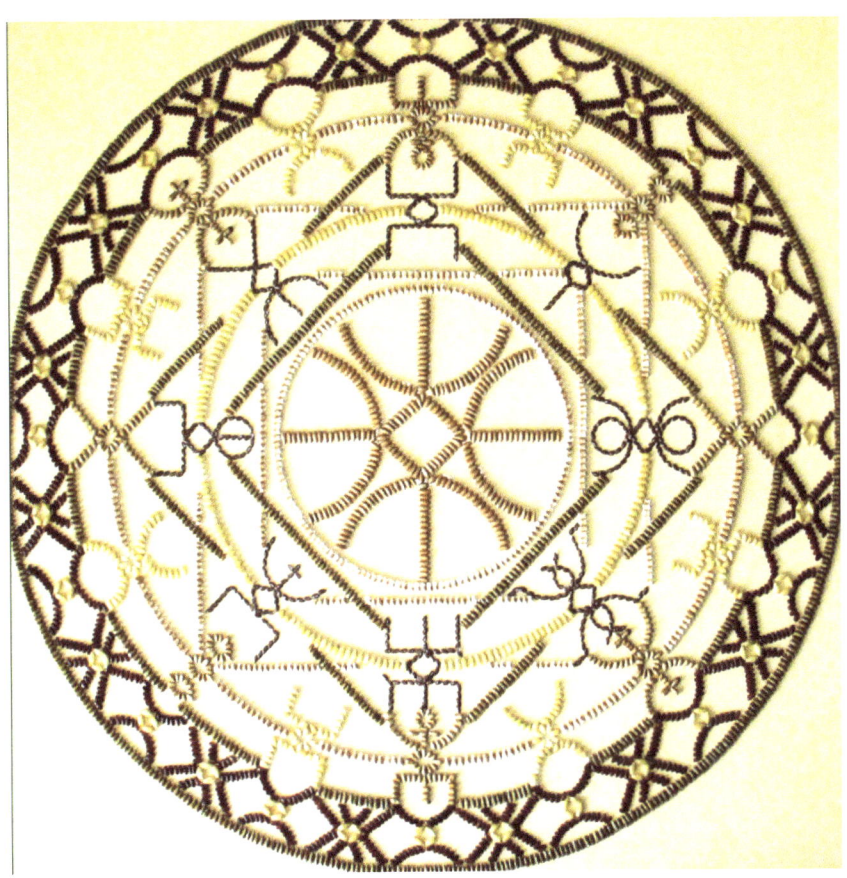

Illustration 3. *Universal Wealth*
This mandala is a potent activator of those aspects of soul and mind which allow a person to remain wealthy (material and spiritual). It is no secret that the universe is abundant in nature, and the only hurdle that prevents all these benefits is in the person himself. This mandala will help not only to get rid of non-structural systems, but also to attract into your life more external opportunities and resources.

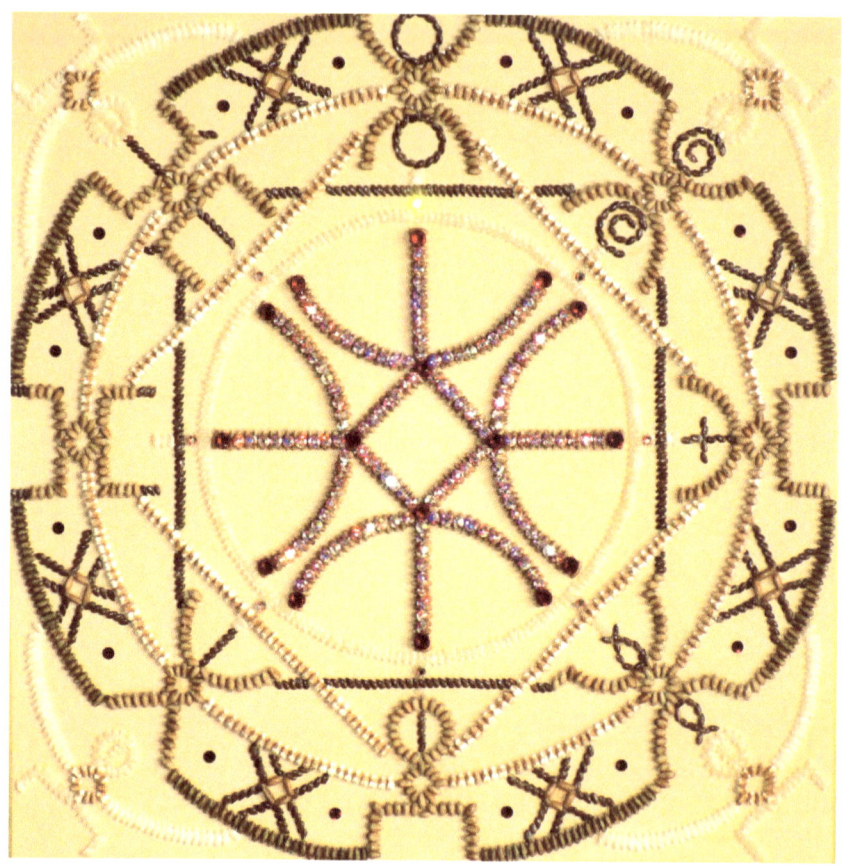

Illustration 4. *Universal Prosperity (small)*
This mandala was created in order to tune our psyche to that primary state
of prosperity, from which the deep financial rivers and well-equipped
material banks originate. It is important to realize that the growth and
development do not come from trauma, but out of a sense of completeness.
All wisdom, wealth and beauty of the universe are in the person himself, one
only need to activate them.

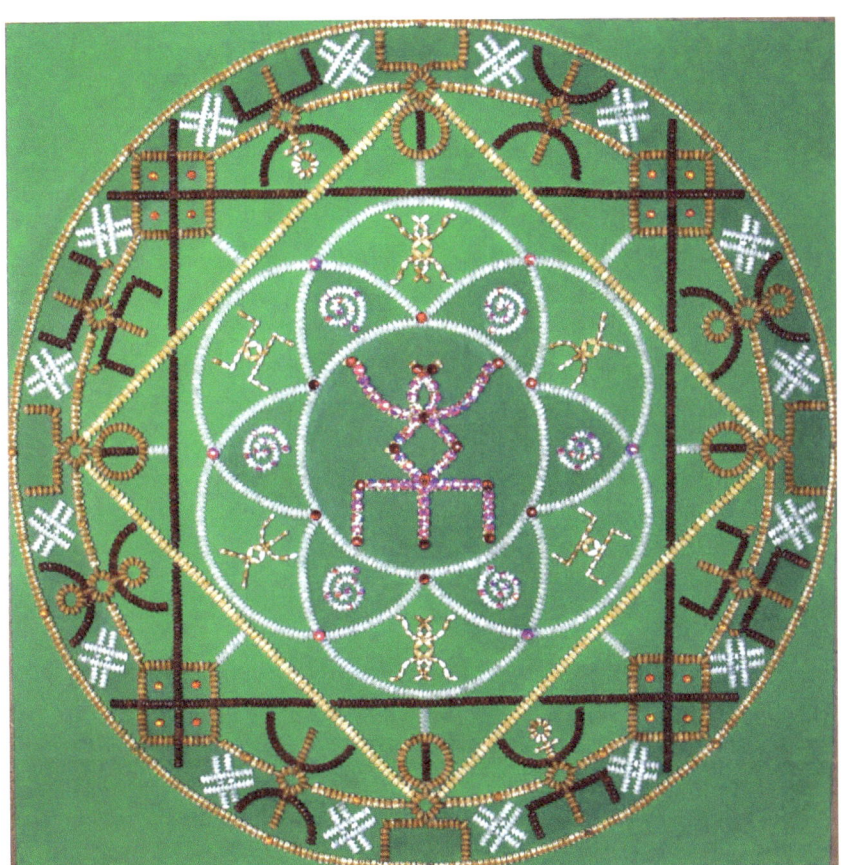

Illustration 5. *"Healer"*
This mandala is dedicated to the main "doctor" of the Slavic rune row - the "Restorer" rune. The structure of this rune combines two principles: purification and love. Cleansing helps to remove the effects of trauma and destructive programs, and love heals mental wounds. Mandala contributes to the fastest possible restoration of the body and soul of a person, and, as a result, success in his life path.

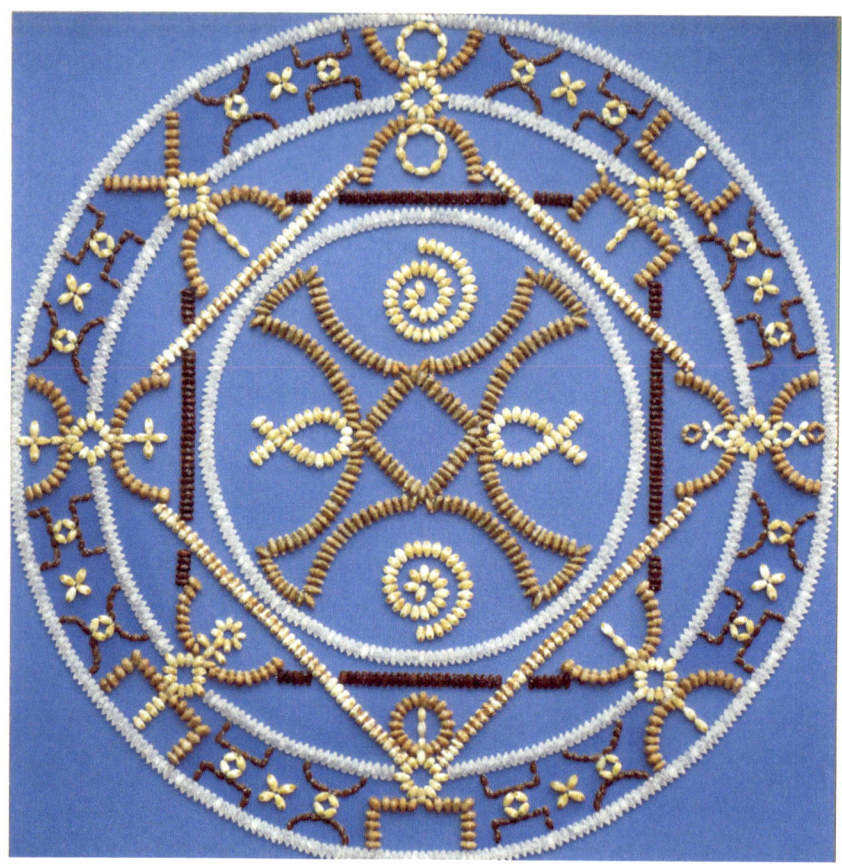

Illustration 6. *Whirlwind of Love*

This mandala was created to open the paths of love. It can be of invaluable support in those situations where a person experiences constant difficulties in interpersonal relationships and cannot understand the reasons for these. In the center of this mandala are the runes Love and Whirlwind. The whirlwind, in this case, helps not only to "blow out" the obstacles, but also to bring consciousness to the origins of the problem.

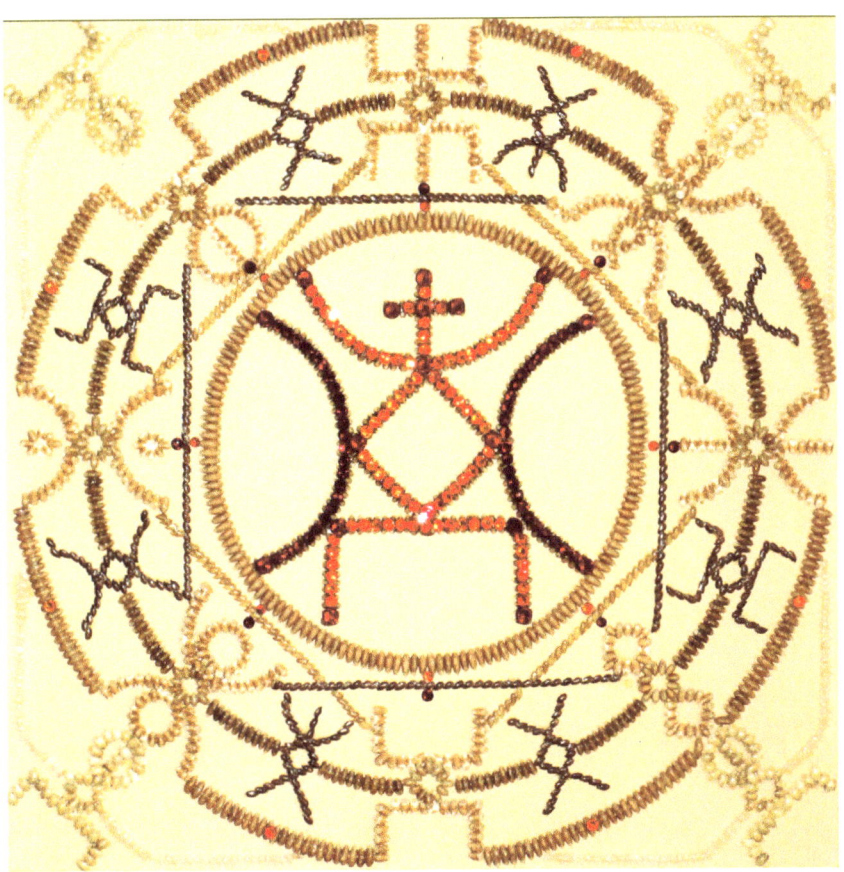

Illustration 7. *Victory Path*
This mandala carries the solar masculine energy of victory. This is the mandala of success. The central runes Path and Victory will help a person achieve his plan, realize his strengths and weaknesses, remain in the stream with life and follow the path of his destiny.

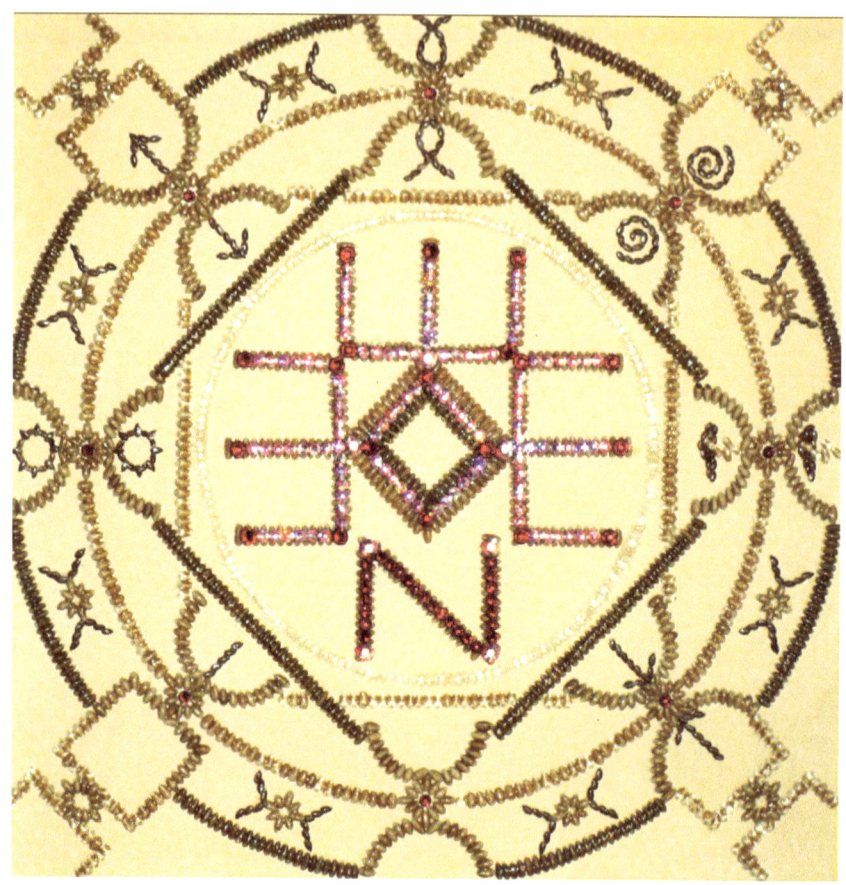

Illustration 8. *Cleansing and Getting Rid of Lies*
This mandala helps to overcome the widest range of manipulations
(energetic, informational, emotional, etc.). It cleans the human field from
destructive programs and harmful mental images. It is especially useful for
those who work with people or are often forced to be in places where people
quarrel or get sick. By cutting off the energy "parasites", it returns to the
person his original power.

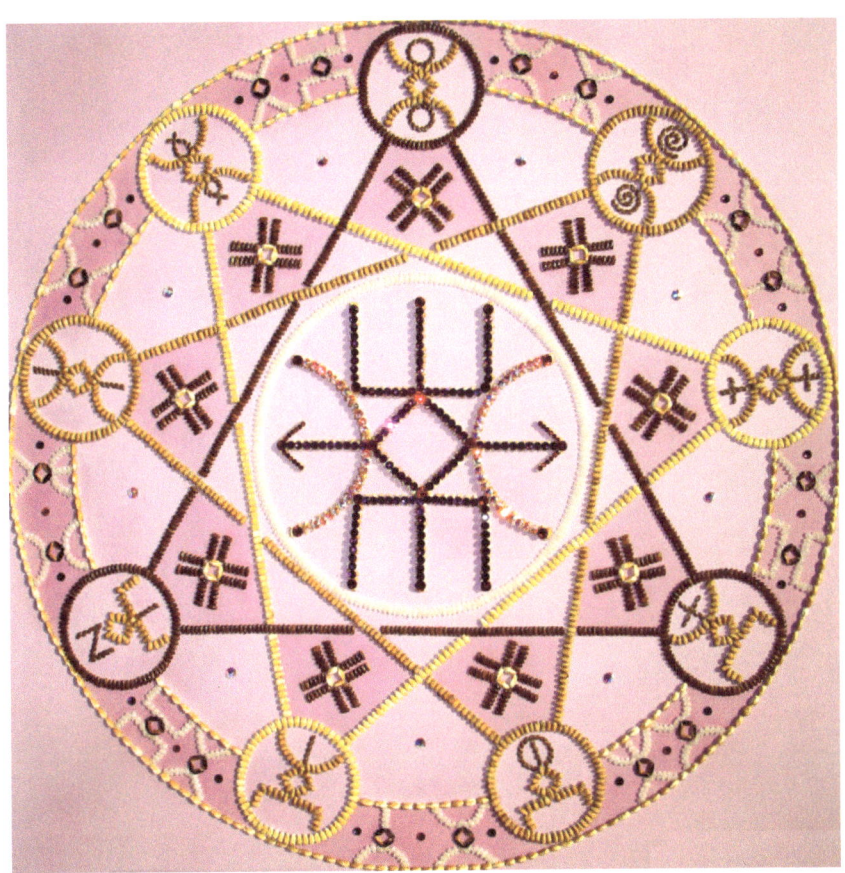

Illustration 9. *Purification and Scattering*

This mandala helps to cleanse and dissipate the destructive energies and barriers that a person encounter on the way to his goals. It helps transform obstacles into vital resources by resolving any problem constructively. The essence of this mandala is to take the force from the foe and wrap it up for your own good.

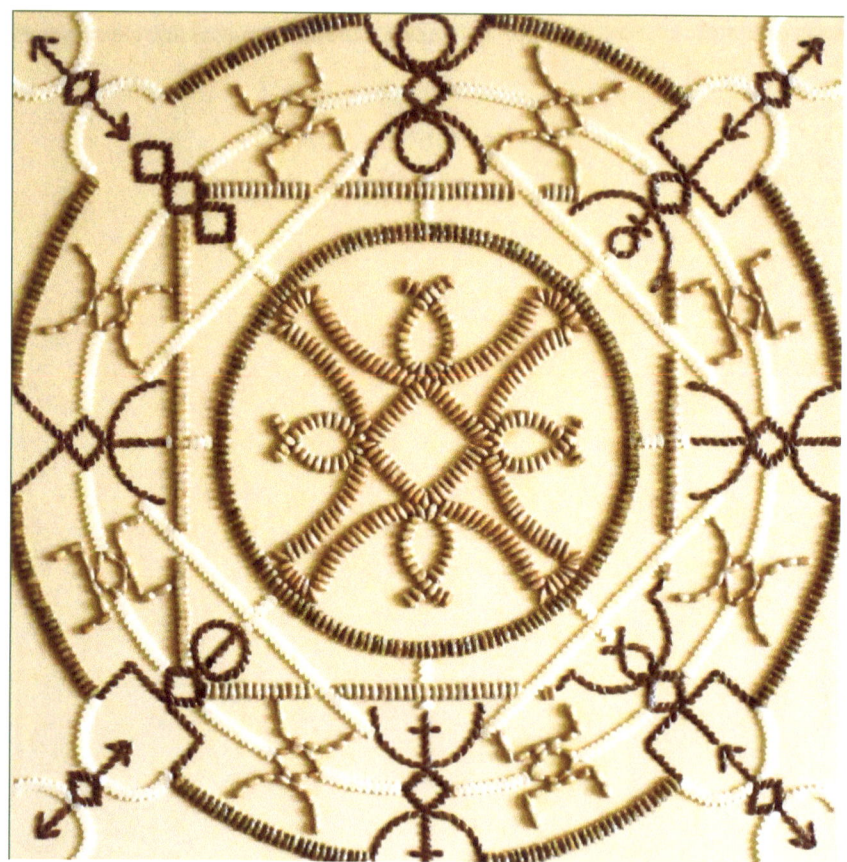

Illustration 10. *Universal Love*

This mandala is a potent activator of love in the broadest sense of the word. It will help not only to get rid of the resentment and, thus, upgrade the existing relationships, but also to attract into one's life events and people "in tune" to the person. Its practice will reveal a healthy sense of altruism and generosity, along with filling the surrounding space with love!

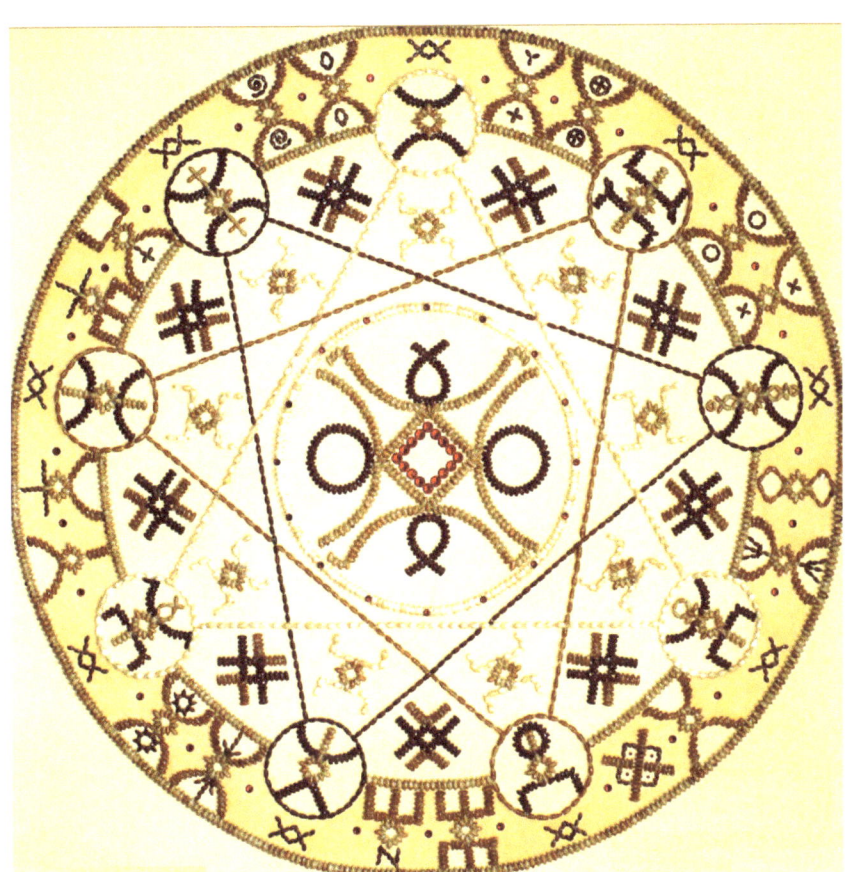

Illustration 11. *Love and Balance*
This mandala carries the "structure" of the protector of the family. The central runes Love and Balance fill a person with feminine energies of unconditional love and acceptance of reality as it is. Both energies, being inscribed in the star of Iglia (a symbol that harmonizes the inner with the outer), are multiplied and fill the space around with light and comfort that only a sincerely loving woman can create.

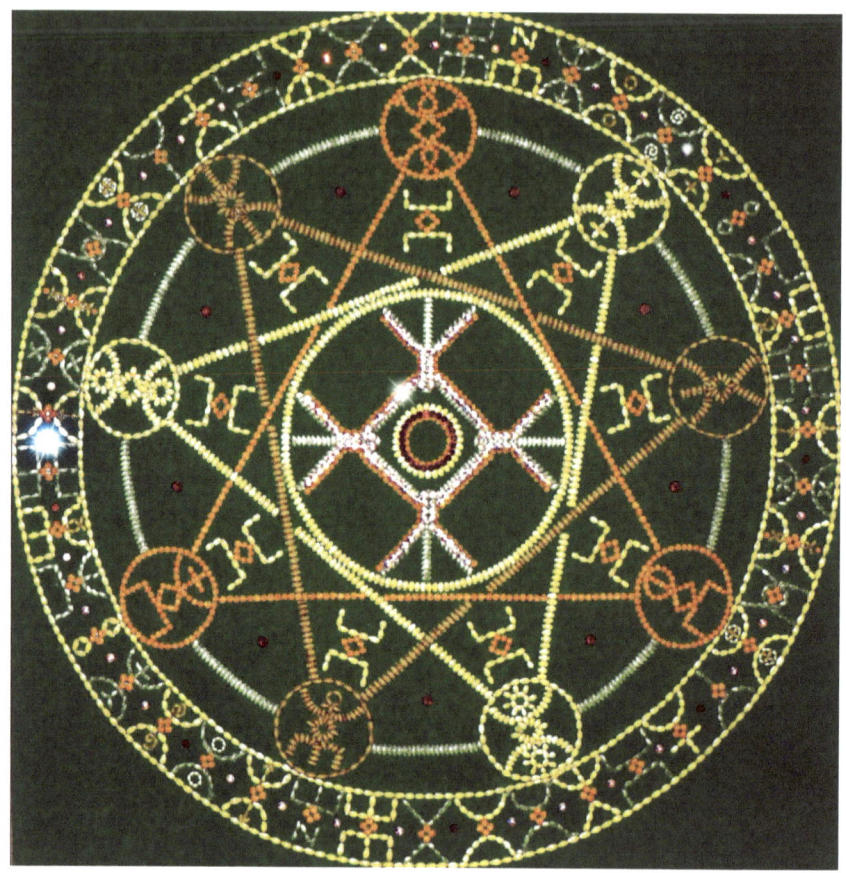

Illustration 12. *Glory*
The mandala carries the energies of two symbols significantly valued in the Slavic-Aryan tradition: the Slav rune and the star of Iglia. Glory symbolizes the world of glorious ancestors-heroes, guardians and defenders of the family. The mandala is beneficial to a person who sets big goals for himself. Glory helps to achieve success and respect in society in the path of a person's true destiny. Being inscribed in the star of Iglia (a symbol that harmonizes the inner with the outer), Glory is greatly enhanced.

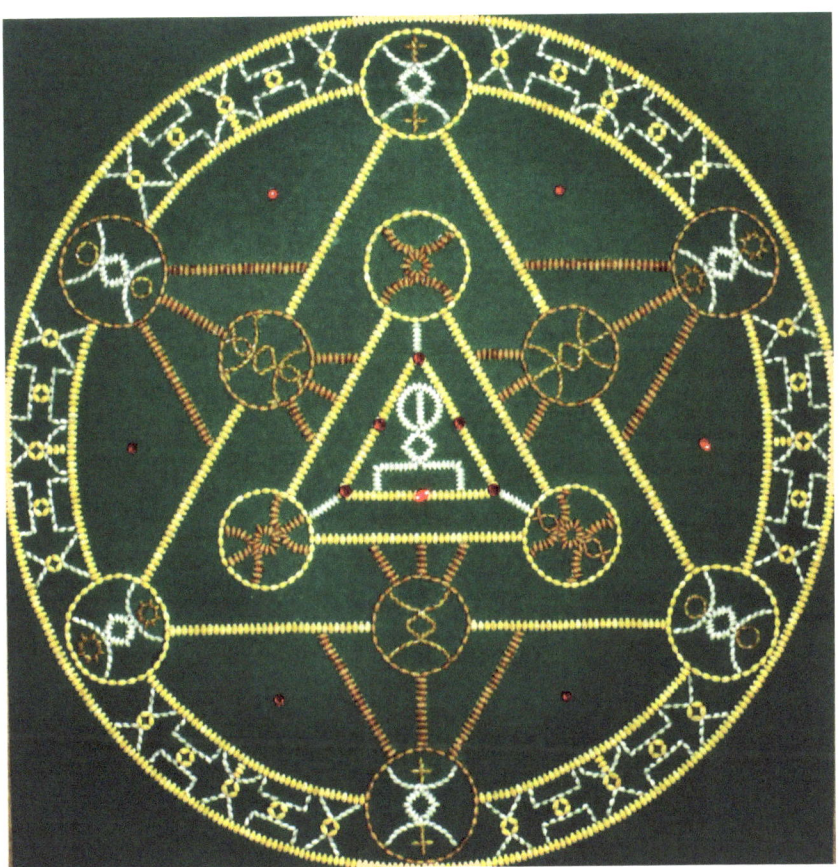

Illustration 13. *Growth*

This mandala is beneficial for a person who feels that the time has come to change something in life. This mandala in all its forms symbolizes growth. It represents the energy of the spring sun and energy of life, which even sprout the grass beneath asphalt. The structure of the mandala contains the strongest sacred symbol Mer-ka-ba, sometimes also called the Flower of Life. It symbolizes absolute harmony, the fusion of spirit and soul.

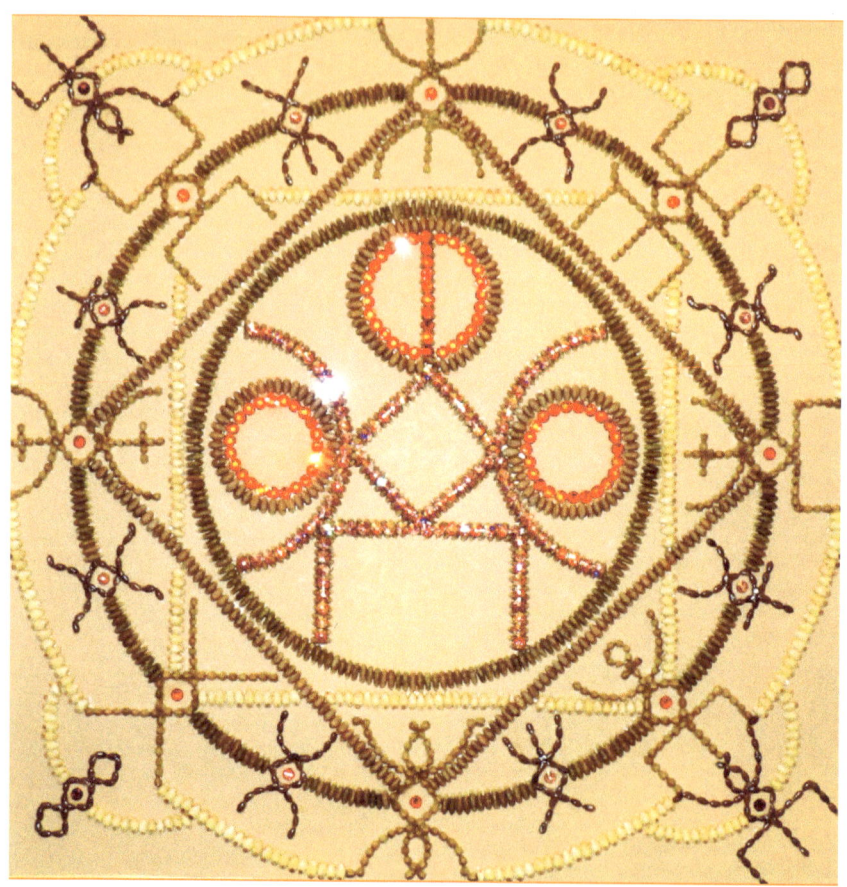

Illustration 14. *Equilibrium Growth*

This mandala brings harmony and balance to the outer and inner space of a person. The two central Slavic runes "Growth" and "Equilibrium" contribute to balancing various aspects of life, along with gently removing "imbalances", such as fixation at work, relationships, finances, etc.

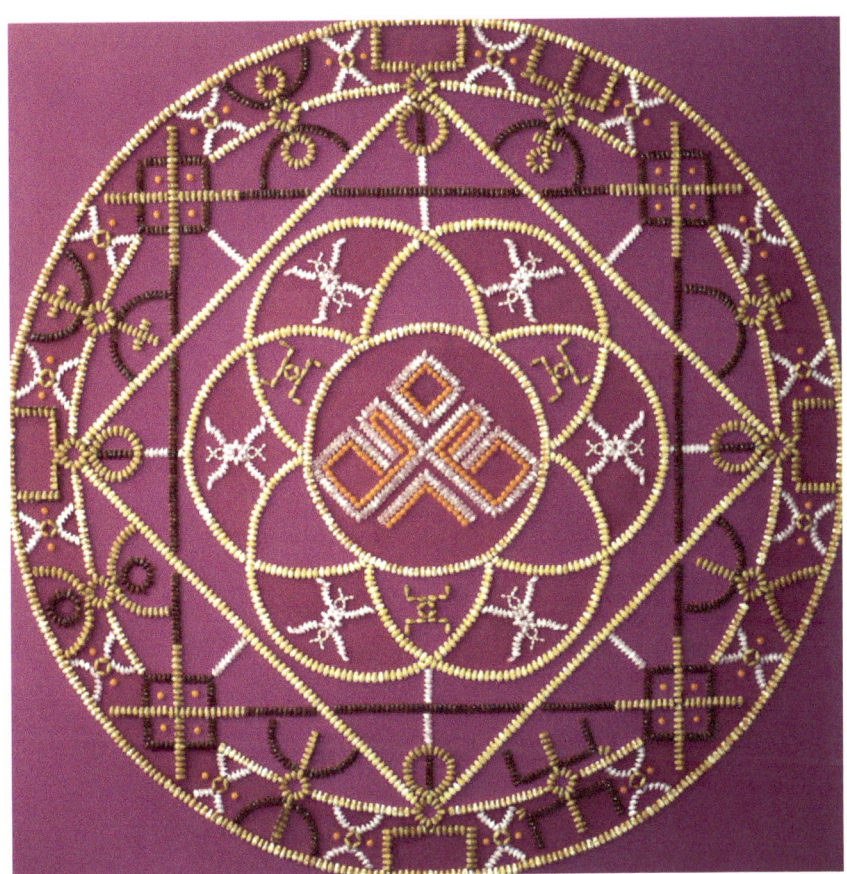

Illustration 15. *Feminine Fertility Energy*

This mandala carries the energy of Rozhanitsa - the Slavic Goddess, personifying the female life-giving principle and the great mystery of Nature, symbolizing female fertility. The mandala symbolizes all key manifestations of feminine energy. Both pregnant women and those who could not get pregnant often turn to this symbol for help.

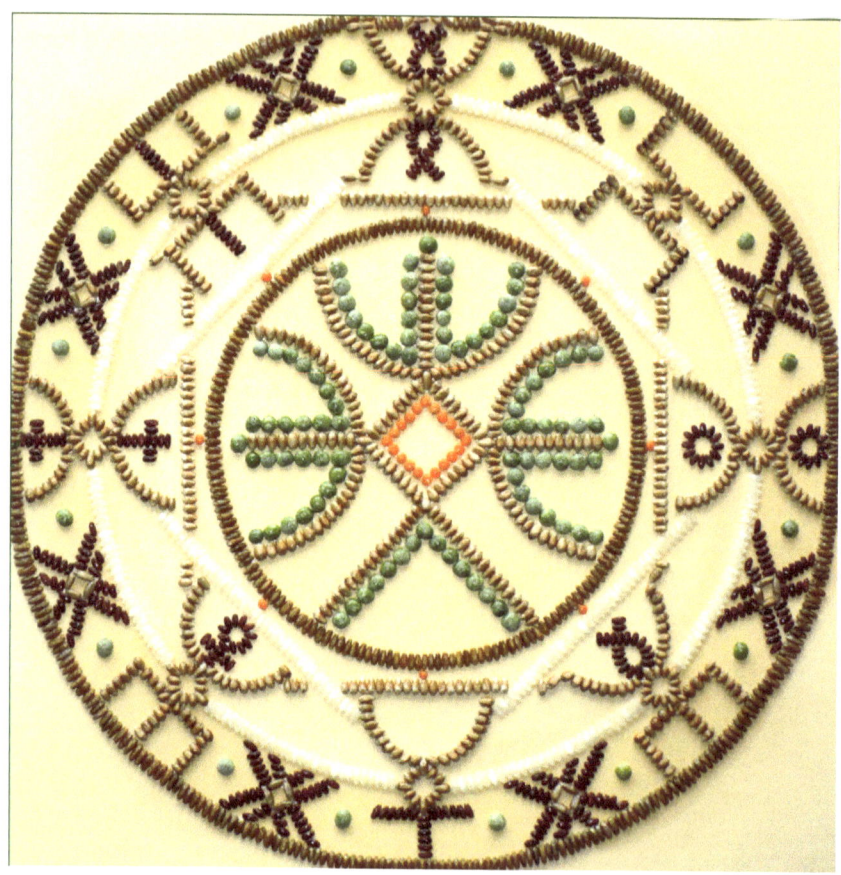

Illustration 16. *Plenty of Joy*
Somewhere very deep inside each of us sits a child who was once innocent
and free. This mandala helps to find a child inside us and to return to
ourselves not only the joy of creativity, which this little one holds in his
hands, but also the joy of life in general. It helps to realize that the joy does
not live in the achievements of life, but lives in the soul and body.

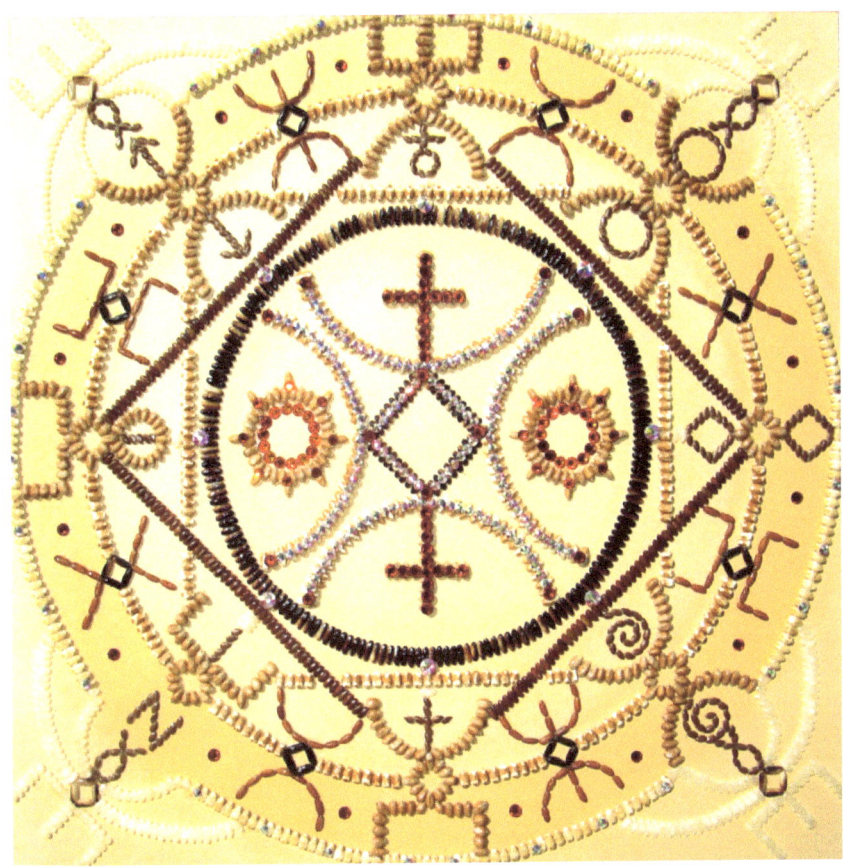

Illustration 17. *Clear Knowledge*
This is the mandala of intuition, deep knowledge of the whole and disclosure of "beyond the abilities" of a person. In the center are two Slavic runes "Vision" and "Clarity". Both of these runes are aimed at gaining true multi-level knowledge about people, events, nature of things, motives for actions, etc. The mandala allows one to use this knowledge for the benefit of oneself and universe.

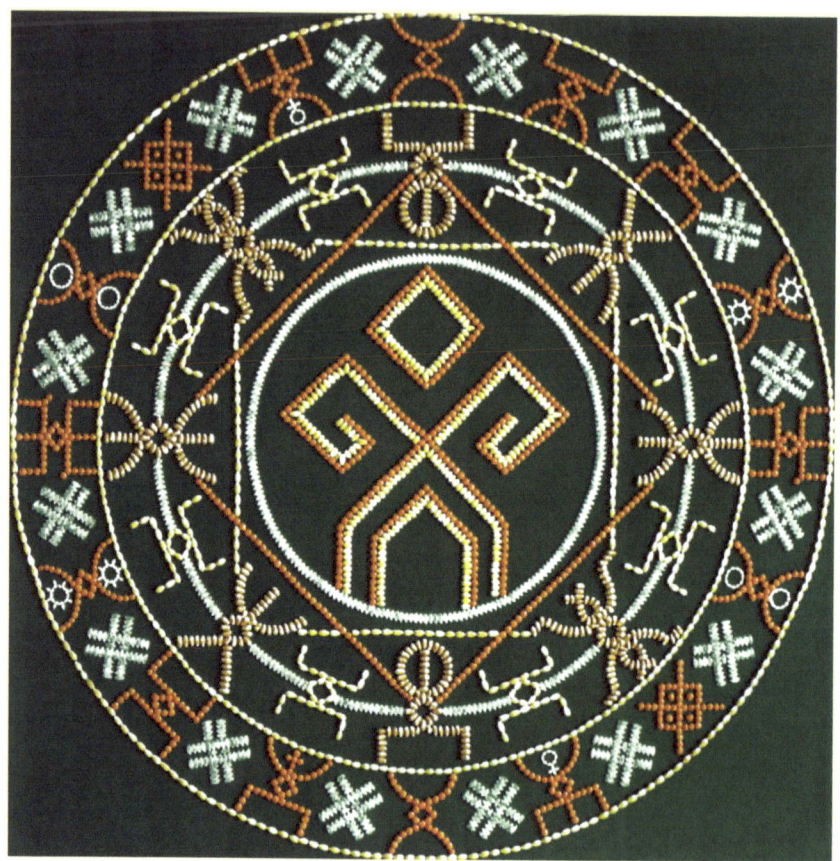

Illustration 18. *Chur (Ancestral House Defender)*
This mandala is dedicated to the most revered in the Slavic tradition: the
ancestral protector of the family and house - Chur. Chur is considered the
keeper of light on earth, while the sun is in the sky. A charm with the image
of Chur used to be placed in the house, and our ancestors believed that no
evil would enter the house as long as Chur "the protector" took care of it.

CPSIA information can be obtained
at www.ICGtesting.com
Printed in the USA
BVHW020952060421
604323BV00012B/150